Endoscopic Diagnosis of the Female Lower Urinary Tract

Commissioning Editor: Miranda Bromage
Development Editor: Rachel Robson
Project Supervisor: Mark Sanderson
Typeset by Paston PrePress Ltd, Beccles, Suffolk
Printed in Hong Kong

Endoscopic Diagnosis of the Female Lower Urinary Tract

by

Geoffrey W. Cundiff BA MD FACOG
Assistant Professor, Director of Gynecologic Endoscopy,
Duke University Medical Center,
Division of Gynecologic Specialities,
Durham, North Carolina, USA

and

Alfred E. Bent MD
Head, Division of Urogynecology/Reconstructive Pelvic Surgery,
Greater Baltimore Medical Center,
Baltimore, Maryland, USA

W. B. Saunders

London • Edinburgh • New York • Philadelphia • Sydney • Toronto

W. B. SAUNDERS
A Division of Harcourt Brace and Company Limited

ISBN 0-7020-2352-3

First published 1999

British Library Cataloguing in Publication Data
A catalogue record for this book is available from the British Library

Library of Congress Cataloging in Publication Data
A catalog record for this book is available from the Library of Congress

Medical knowledge is constantly changing. As new information becomes available,
changes in treatment, procedures, equipment and the use of drugs become necessary.
The authors and Publishers have, as far as it is possible, taken care to ensure that the
information given in the text is accurate and up to date. However, readers are strongly
advised to confirm that the information, especially with regard to drug usage, complies
with latest legislation and standards of practice.

The
Publisher's
policy is to use
**paper manufactured
from sustainable forests**

Table of Contents

Acknowledgements

We gratefully acknowledge the contribution of Karl Storz Endoscopy – America, Inc., Culver City, California, USA for providing equipment to facilitate photodocumentation.

Additionally, we would like to recognize our colleagues, Rick Bump and Glenn Hart for their important contributions to the concept of this book.

Dedication

The authors wish to dedicate this textbook to Jack R. Robertson, M.D. He made significant contributions in defining urethroscopy, especially for the gynecologist and produced some of the first and finest high quality color photographs of pathology in the female bladder and urethra. He has contributed to urogynecology nationally and internationally for over 30 years. His use of carbon dioxide for urethroscopy and the cystometrogram became the standard to which other techniques were compared for years.

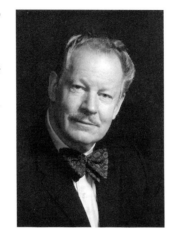

Appreciation

To my wife, Callie, who is the real photographer in the family, and has documented our travels so expertly; thanks for your patience and continued encouragement in my chosen profession.

Alfred E. Bent

And to my wife, Valerie, who has been gracious and sincere in her support of this project as in all my professional endeavors.

Geoffrey W. Cundiff

Table of Figures by Chapter

·CHAPTER 1

Historical perspective

Geoffrey W. Cundiff

EARLY CYSTOSCOPES

Kelly is frequently credited with the development of the female cystoscope, and yet endoscopy of the female bladder preceded his report by nearly a century. In 1805, Bozzini[1] designed a lichtleiter consisting of a stand that supported differently sized hollow funnels, a candle for illumination, and a reflector to direct the light into the funnel when it was placed into the urethra. He used the endoscope in cadavers and several live patients evaluating the vagina, rectum, an abdominal incision, and, in one woman, the urethra and bladder. While Bozzini's endoscope did not provide adequate illumination, it did have potential. Regrettably, the far from innovative Medical Faculty of Vienna squashed the invention before it could be developed more fully.[2]

NINETEENTH-CENTURY INNOVATIONS

Desormeaux, sometimes cited as the father of cystoscopy, introduced a more practical endoscope to the French Academy of Medicine in Paris in 1853.[3] His device used an angled viewing tube at a right angle to the light source (Fig. 1.1). While he initially used a candle as a light source, he significantly improved illumination by switching to an alcohol lamp and later to camphor with petroleum to increase the

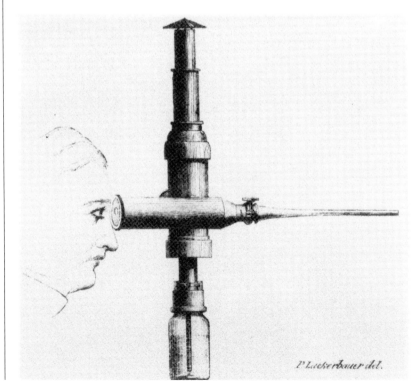

Fig. 1.1 Desormeaux's cystoscope

light from the flame. Visibility with this device was limited both by the narrow viewing tube and the tendency of operators to burn themselves if the device was tilted for a better view. Segalas introduced an outer cannula to the endoscope, which facilitated introduction of the endoscope into the urethra. He also added reflective mirrors to improve illumination.[4]

Grünfeld further modified the cystoscope in 1877.[5] His cystoscope still utilized a hollow tube, but with a glass lens placed obliquely at the distal end. This allowed for a larger field of vision, but at the expense of an inverted image. The early cystoscopists who used cystoscopes with a lens had to compensate for this inversion in maneuvering the cystoscope within the bladder. This inconvenience was finally overcome thirty years later by the introduction of a prism into the telescope.[6]

An adequate light source continued to elude the early endoscopists. Even with the use of a compound lens and reflective mirrors, illumination was not ideal. The introduction of electricity provided new opportunities to improve illumination. In 1867, Bruck proposed transillumination of the bladder for cystoscopy.[7] This was accomplished by using a powerful incandescent platinum wire placed in the rectum to transilluminate the bladder base. Unfortunately, this was insufficient light and, even with water cooling, rectal burns occurred.

Nitze is often credited with developing modern cystoscopy. In 1879, he combined the platinum wire of Bruck's endoscope with a compound lens system. All previous innovations to improve illumination used an external light source reflected into the bladder.[8] The unique aspect of Nitze's cystoscope was the introduction of the light source into the bladder cavity. While this provided an excellent light source, it required irrigation of the bladder with cold water to prevent burns. Nitze made further innovations with instrument maker Joseph Leiter (Fig. 1.2). In 1887, using Edison's invention of the incandescent light bulb, they presented an instrument that no longer needed cooling irrigation.[7] Nitze also constructed a urethral and operating cystoscope, but, more importantly, made numerous observations of normal and pathologic findings which were described in his *Textbook of Cystoscopy* first published in 1889.[9] In spite of his many contributions to cystoscopy, Nitze's cystoscope was considered to be too complicated for all but the specialist.

In 1889, Boisseau de Rocher developed an outer sheath separate from the ocular portion of the cystoscope, which made it possible to use multiple telescopes within a single sheath. This simplified operative manipulation, as is illustrated by Poirer's report that year

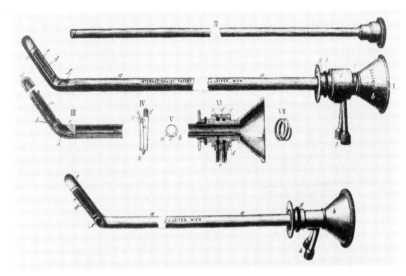

Fig. 1.2 Nitze–Leiter cystoscope.
a. Telescope sheath; **b.** eyepiece; **c.** blunt
end; **d.** light source fenestration;
e. platinum wire; **f.** distal lens

of successfully catheterizing both ureters in a living patient using this instrumentation.[4]

Even with these improvements in the cystoscope and illumination, visualization was still poor without bladder distension. Additionally, acquiring and servicing cystoscopic equipment was difficult for American physicians, as it was largely manufactured in Europe. By the end of the nineteenth century, most physicians considered cystoscopy to be nothing more than an adjunct to the established method of urethral dilation followed by bimanual palpation.

THE KELLY CYSTOSCOPE

Kelly's contribution to cystoscopy was in developing a technique that overcame the deficiencies of the nineteenth-century instruments.[10] The Kelly cystoscope (Fig. 1.3), a hollow tube or speculum without a

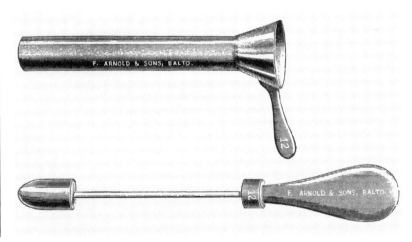

Fig. 1.3 Kelly's cystoscope

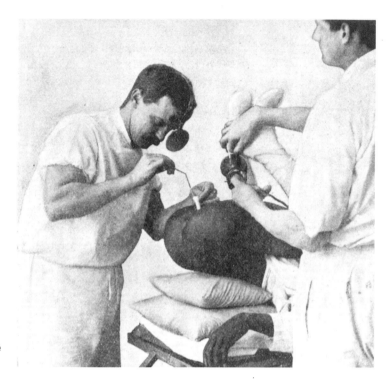

Fig. 1.4 Kelly's technique of air cystoscopy. The patient's hips are in extreme elevation, and Kelly uses a probe to find the ureteral orifice with light directed from the held light source into the bladder using a head mirror

lens, was not innovative, but his technique was. The cystoscope was introduced using an obturator, with the patient's hips in extreme elevation. In this position, introduction of the cystoscope allowed air to distend the bladder. A head mirror was used to reflect an electric light into the bladder for illumination. The technique was simple yet provided an excellent view. Kelly was also the first to pass ureteral catheters under direct vision. His technique for direct catheterization of the ureters was also performed with the patient positioned with hips in moderate elevation (Fig. 1.4).

The simplicity of air cystoscopy made cystoscopy available to all physicians for the first time. Kelly's fame as a genitourinary surgeon, and as the founder of the Johns Hopkins Hospital residency training program in gynecology – the first in the nation – established cystoscopy as a gynecologic technique.

ROD LENS CYSTOSCOPES

The introduction of the Hopkins' fiberoptic telescope in 1954 marked the beginning of modern cystoscopy.[11] The use of glass fibers in place of an air chamber dramatically improved light transmission and resolution. It also provided a wider viewing field, and permitted a change in the viewing angle. The innovation of angled telescopes improved the extent of visualization and facilitated more invasive

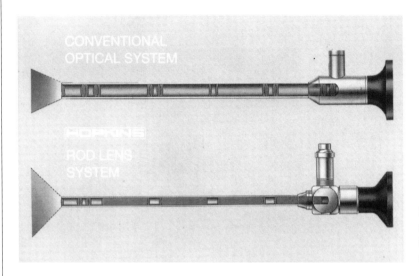

Fig. 1.5 Hopkins rod lens system. (Reproduced with permission from Karl Storz Endoscopy, Culver City, California, USA)

procedures. The glass fibers were subsequently replaced by a series of glass rods with optically finished ends, separated by intervening spaces (Fig. 1.5). This rod lens design is the system used in today's rigid cystoscopes.

The use of a series of glass rods with optically finished ends, separated by intervening air spaces, provides excellent resolution with a wider viewing field, and permits a change in the viewing angle. The innovation of angled telescopes improved the extent of visualization and facilitated more invasive procedures. Increasingly complex instruments were developed to perform operative procedures through a cystoscope, and gradually general surgeons developed the subspecialty of urology around this new technology. The development of the subspecialty of urology coincident with the combination of gynecology and obstetrics into a single training program de-emphasized cystoscopy in gynecologic training, and gynecologists gradually became less skilled with the technique.

ROBERTSON URETHROSCOPE

The illumination and angled view of the Hopkins cystoscope used with a closed irrigation system provided an excellent view of the entire bladder wall but was not ideal for viewing the urethra. The deflected field of view of an angled cystoscope does not permit straight-on viewing of the urethral lumen unless the entire cystoscope is angled, which distorts the axis of the lumen. Additionally, the terminal fenestra of the traditional cystoscope sheath allows the irrigant to escape during viewing of the distal urethra and this prevents adequate distension of the lumen. Robertson addressed the deficiencies of the cystoscope for viewing the urethra by applying the rod lens technology of the Hopkins cystoscope to a shorter straight-on telescope with a non-fenestrated sheath, designed specifically for viewing the urethra.[12] As the father of urogynecology, Robertson's development of the urethroscope reintroduced cystoscopy to gynecology.

Robertson subsequently outlined a technique, dynamic urethroscopy, for evaluating incontinent women using the Robertson urethroscope. Dynamic urethroscopy offered a simple office procedure that considerably improved the diagnostic evaluation of the lower urinary tract. This technique is more fully described in Chapter 3.

FLEXIBLE CYSTOSCOPES

The most recent development in cystoscopy is the flexible cystoscope. A flexible cystoscope takes advantage of the flexibility of the fiberoptic lens system to create a cystoscope that bends, thereby increasing the range of the field of view. Tsuchida and Sugawara[13] reported an improved view of the bladder neck utilizing a flexible fiber cystoscope. Others have advocated flexible cystoscopy as a means to limit the necessary instrumentation and improve patient tolerance.[14]

CONCLUSION

The progressive evolution of instrumentation and techniques over the last two centuries has provided today's pelvic surgeon with the ability to visualize the female lower urinary tract for both diagnostic and operative ends.

REFERENCES

1. Bozzini P. Lichteiter, eine erfindung zur anschung innerer theile, und krukheiten nebst abbildung. *J Pract Arzeykunde* 1805; **24**: 107.
2. Schutte H, Herman JR. Philipp Bozzini (1773–1809). *Invest Urol* 1972; **9**: 447–8.
3. Desnos E. The nineteenth century. In Murphy LJT (ed.) *The History of Urology*. Springfield: Charles C Thomas, 1972: 152–87.
4. Rosenzweig BA. Endoscopic evaluation of the lower urinary tract. In Walters MD, Karram MM (eds) *Clinical Urogynecology*. St Louis: Mosby, 1993, 124–33.
5. Grünfeld. *Der Harnröhrenspiegel (das Endoscop), seine diagnostische und therapeutische Anwendung*. Vienna, 1877.
6. Nicholson P. Problems encountered by early endoscopists. *Urology* 1982; **19**: 114–19.
7. Rathert P. Max Nitze (1848–1906). *Invest Urol* 1967; **5**: 327–30.
8. Nitze M. Eine neue balbachtungs-und untersuchunigsmethods fur harnrohre, harnbiase und rectum. *Wein Med Wochenschr* 1879; **24**: 649.
9. Nitze M. *Lehrbruch der Kystoskopie*. Wiesbaden, 1889.
10. Kelly HA. The direct examination of the female bladder with elevated pelvis – the catheterization of the ureters under direct inspection, with and without elevation of

the pelvis. *American Journal of Obstetrics and Diseases of Women and Children* 1894; **29**: 1–19.

11. Hopkins HH, Kopany NS. A flexible fiberscope, using static scanning. *Nature* 1954; **179**: 39–41.

12. Robertson JR. Air cystoscopy. *Obstet Gynecol* 1968; **32**: 328.

13. Tsuchida S, Sugawara H. A new flexible fibercystoscope for visualization of the bladder neck. *J Urol* 1973; **91**: 830.

14. Kavoussi LR, Clayman RV. Office flexible cystoscopy. *Urol Clin North Am* 1988; **15**: 601–8.

CHAPTER 2

Instrumentation for cystourethroscopy

Geoffrey W. Cundiff

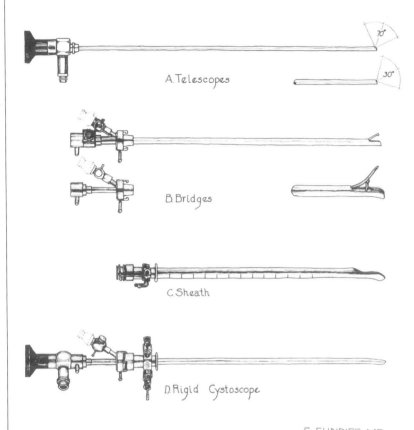

G. CUNDIFF MD

Fig. 2.1 Components of a rigid cystoscope. **a.** Telescopes, 30° and 70°; **b.** bridges, operative and Albarran; **c.** sheath; **d.** assembled cystoscope

RIGID CYSTOSCOPY

The rigid cystoscope is comprised of three parts: the telescope, the bridge, and the sheath (Fig. 2.1). Each component serves a different function and is available with various options to facilitate its role.

Telescope

The telescope transmits light to the bladder cavity as well as an image to the viewer. Today, virtually all rigid telescopes use a rod lens system. Telescopes designed for cystoscopy are available with several viewing angles (Fig. 2.2) including 0° (straight), 30° (forward-oblique), 70° (lateral), and 120° (retroview). The angled telescopes have a field marker that helps maintain orientation. The marker is visible as a blackened notch at the outside of the visual field and opposite the angle of deflection.

The different angles facilitate the inspection of the entire bladder wall. Although the 0° lens is essential for adequate urethroscopy, it is insufficient for cystoscopy. The 30° lens provides the best view of the

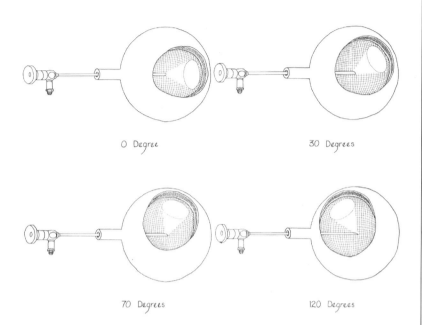

O Degree   30 Degrees

70 Degrees   120 Degrees

Fig. 2.2 Angled telescopes

bladder base and posterior wall, while the 70° lens permits inspection of the anterolateral walls. The retroview of the 120° lens is not usually necessary for cystoscopy of the female bladder but can be useful for evaluating the urethral opening into the bladder. For many applications, a single telescope is preferable. In diagnostic cystoscopy, the 30° telescope usually is sufficient although a 70° telescope may be required in the presence of fixation of the urethrovesical junction. For operative cystoscopy, the 70° telescope is preferable.

Sheath

The cystoscope sheath provides a vehicle for introducing the telescope and distending media into the vesical cavity. Sheaths are available in various calibers ranging from 17 to 28F. When placed within the sheath, the telescope, which is 15F, fills the lumen only partially, leaving an irrigation–working channel. The smallest diameter sheath is useful for diagnostic procedures while the larger calibers provide space for the placement of instruments into the irrigation–working channel. The proximal end of the sheath has two irrigating ports, one for introduction of the distending media and another for its exit. The distal end of the cystoscope sheath is fenestrated to permit use of instrumentation in the angled field of view. It is also beveled, opposite the fenestration, to increase the comfort of introduction of the cystoscope into the urethra. Bevels increase with the diameter of the cystoscope and larger diameter sheaths may require an obturator for placement.

Bridge

The bridge serves as a connector between the telescope and sheath, and forms a water-tight seal with both. It may also have one or two ports for introduction of instruments into the irrigation–working channel. The Albarran bridge is a variation of the bridge originally designed for an operative version of the Nitze telescope of the late nineteenth century. It has a deflector mechanism located at the distal end of the inner sheath. When placed within the cystoscope sheath, the deflector mechanism is located at the distal end of the inner sheath within the fenestration of the outer sheath. In this location, elevation of the deflector mechanism assists the manipulation of instruments within the field of view (Fig. 2.1b).

FLEXIBLE CYSTOSCOPY

Unlike the rigid cystoscope, the flexible cystoscope combines the optical systems and irrigation–working channel in a single unit. The optical system consists of a single image-bearing fiberoptic bundle and two light-bearing fiberoptic bundles. The fibers of these bundles are coated parallel coherent optical fibers that transmit light even when bent. This permits incorporation of a distal tip-deflecting mechanism that will deflect the tip 290° in a single plane. The deflection is controlled by a lever at the eyepiece. The optical fibers are fitted to a lens system that magnifies and focuses the image. A focusing knob is located just distal to the eyepiece. The irrigation–working port enters the instrument at the eyepiece opposite the deflecting mechanism. The coated tip is 15–18F in diameter and 6–7 cm in length, with the working unit comprising half the length (Fig. 2.3).

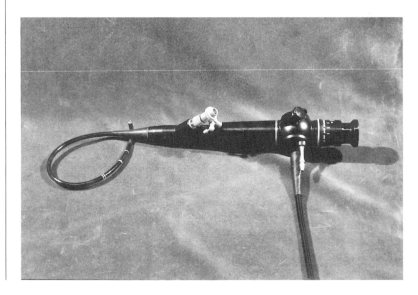

Fig. 2.3 Flexible cystourethroscope

Because of the individual coating of the fibers there is a small space between each fiber in the image guide. Consequently, the image appears somewhat granular. The delicate 5–10-μm diameter of the fibers makes them susceptible to damage which will further compromise the image or light transmission. Gentle handling is, therefore, essential to good visualization, not to mention the longevity of the instrument. The flow rate of the irrigation–working channel is approximately one fourth that of a similarly sized rigid cystoscope and is further curtailed by passage of instruments down this channel. Some tip deflection is also lost with use of the instrument channel.

In spite of these restrictions, several studies have compared rigid with flexible cystoscopy and found no compromise of diagnostic capabilities.[1,2] Many urologists prefer the flexible cystoscope because of improved patient comfort, but the improved comfort applies primarily to male patients who often require general anesthesia for diagnostic cystoscopy with a rigid instrument. The absence of a prostate and the short length of the female urethra make rigid cystoscopy well tolerated by women. This may offset any perceived advantage of flexible cystoscopy in female patients.

RIGID URETHROSCOPY

The rigid urethroscope has two components (Fig. 2.4), the sheath and the telescope. The telescope transmits light to the end of the telescope

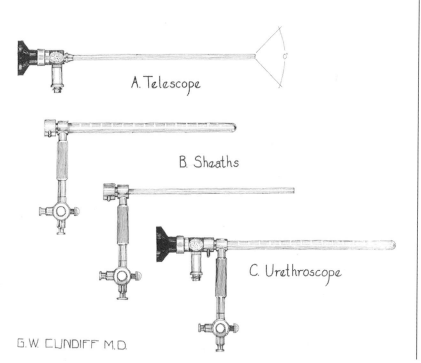

Fig. 2.4 Components of a rigid urethroscope. **a.** Telescopes, 0°; **b.** sheaths, 15 and 24F; **c.** assembled urethroscope

G.W. CUNDIFF M.D.

as well as an image to the viewer. Telescopes designed for urethroscopy have a $0°$ viewing angle (straight). This straight-on view provides a circumferential view of the urethral lumen as the mucosa in front of the urethroscope is distended by the distension media. The $0°$ lens is essential to adequate urethroscopy, but is insufficient for cystoscopy.

The urethroscope sheath provides a vehicle for introducing the telescope and distending media into the urethral lumen. The proximal end of the sheath has an irrigating port, for introduction of the distending media. Sheaths are available in 15 and 24F caliber. The largest diameter sheath is useful, if tolerated, as it provides the best view of the urethral lumen by distending it maximally. The telescope only partially fills the sheath, leaving space for the irrigant to flow around it.

LIGHT SOURCES AND VIDEO MONITORS

Any light source that will provide adequate illumination via a fiberoptic cable is sufficient. Many manufacturers have recommended a high-intensity (xenon) light source for the use of video monitoring or photography, although the new cameras now require less light than previous generations.

The cable attaches to the telescope at the eyepiece. Light cables are either fiberoptic or fluid filled. The fluid-filled cables tend to be more expensive and more durable, although they add a slight tint to the light. Fiberoptic cables use flexible optic fibers comparable to those of the flexible cystoscope, and are similarly prone to damage.

Although all cystoscopic procedures can be performed with direct visualization through the eyepiece, video monitoring eliminates the awkward positioning required for direct visualization. It also permits video documentation, which facilitates teaching, and often improves patient toleration by providing distraction during the procedure. The video camera attaches directly to the eyepiece and should be maintained in an upright orientation. Changing the direction of view is accomplished by rotating the cystoscope without moving the camera itself.

DISTENDING MEDIA

Cystourethroscopy has been described with carbon dioxide but most practitioners prefer to use water or saline to distend the bladder and urethra. A liquid medium prevents the carbon dioxide-associated bubbling which can limit visualization, and the bladder volumes achieved using a liquid medium more accurately approximate physiologic volumes. If a liquid medium is utilized, the water is instilled by gravity through a standard intravenous infusion set. The bag should be at a height of at least 100 cm above the patient's pubic symphysis to provide adequate flow.

OPERATIVE INSTRUMENTATION

A wide range of instrumentation is available for use through a cystoscope (Fig. 2.5). Those most pertinent to urogynecology are grasping forceps with either a rat tooth or alligator jaws, biopsy forceps, and scissors. They can be obtained in semi-rigid or flexible varieties and come in various diameters. A flexible monopolar ball electrode (Bugby) is useful for electrocautery but is not essential to operative cystoscopy.

INSTRUMENT CARE

Blood and debris should be removed from the equipment promptly to avoid accumulation in crevices and pitting of metal surfaces. The most common method of sterilization is immersion in a 2% activated glutaraldehyde solution (Cidex; Surgikos, Arlington, Texas, USA). Cystourethroscopic equipment should be soaked for 20 minutes, and then transferred to a basin of sterile water until ready for use. Longer soaks will shorten the life of the telescope by deteriorating the lens system and seals. The Cidex solution is changed once a week, and the sterile water as needed. If more permanent storage is desired, the scopes are cleaned with detergent and water, rinsed and stored. Once

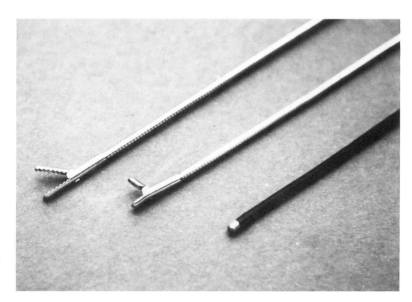

Fig. 2.5 Operative cystoscopic instruments. (Reproduced with permission from Karl Storz Endoscopy, Culver City, California, USA)

a week the scopes are cleaned inside and out with alcohol. The irrigating ports and locking mechanisms should also be lubricated regularly with super oil.

REFERENCES

1. Figueroa TE, Thomas R, Moon TD. A comparison of rigid with flexible instruments. *J La State Med Soc* 1987; **139**: 26.
2. Clayman RV, Reddy P, Lange PH. Flexible fiberoptic and rigid rod lens endoscopy of the lower urinary tract: a prospective controlled comparison. *J Urol* 1984; **131**: 715.

CHAPTER 3

Diagnostic cystourethroscopy

Alfred E. Bent

INDICATIONS AND CONTRAINDICATIONS

Indications for cystourethroscopy include hematuria (gross or microscopic), irritative or obstructive voiding symptoms, recurrent urinary tract infections, incontinence evaluation, interstitial cystitis, foreign body, fistula evaluation, staging for cervical cancer, trauma to the bladder or ureter, urethral diverticulum, and assessment of ureteral function including retrograde studies.[1] It is used early in the diagnosis of potentially serious conditions such as hematuria and fistula, but may be preceded by various therapeutic modalities for many of the other indications. Incontinence evaluation may not always require endoscopy, but the patient with previous failed surgery or a history suggesting intrinsic urethral sphincter deficiency merits this diagnostic technique (Table 3.1).

Contraindications to endoscopy include known acute and subacute infection of the upper or lower urinary tract, or an unstable medical condition requiring urgent management.

EVALUATION OF THE URETHRAL MUCOSA

The large Skene duct openings are seen externally on either side of the urethral meatus (Plate 1.1). The appropriate instrument for evaluating the urethra is a $0°$ telescope with a nonfenestrated sheath, and carbon dioxide or liquid media (see Chapter 2).

The fluid must flow quickly enough to distend the urethra. The urethroscope is placed directly into the distal urethra with the fluid running briskly, and it is advanced slowly to the urethrovesical junction (UVJ) while the urethral lumen is maintained in the center of the field.[2] The normal mucosa in the urethra rolls away from the tip of the urethroscope when the infusion medium is flowing briskly

---

Table 3.1 Indications for cystourethroscopy

Hematuria
Irritative voiding symptoms
Obstructive voiding symptoms
Recurrent urinary tract infections
Interstitial cystitis
Fistula evaluation
Incontinence evaluation
Trauma to lower urinary tract
Urethral or bladder diverticulum
Foreign body
Staging for cervical cancer
Assessment of ureteral function

(Plate 1.2), but falls into place when the flow is stopped (Plate 1.3). A slightly raised area may be seen posteriorly in the center of the urethra, called the urethral crest[3] (Plate 1.4). This is where the longitudinal ureteral muscles continue into the bladder as the superficial trigone, and then proceed down the posterior wall of the urethra as the urethral crest, terminating in a fibrous ring proximal to the external meatus.[4] Subtle furrows of normal mucosa run along either side of the crest giving the urethral mucosa the appearance of longitudinal folds with a comparable vascular pattern.[5] Occasionally a smooth white covering of urethral mucosa is seen, which is squamous metaplasia, a normal physiologic variant (Plate 1.5).

EVALUATION OF THE URETHROVESICAL JUNCTION

After the scope is passed into the bladder, the bladder is filled with fluid while the ureters and trigone are observed. The scope is withdrawn approximately 1 cm distal to the UVJ so it closes one third of the way (Plate 1.6), and the following commands are issued: 'hold your urine' and 'squeeze your rectum'. The normal UVJ closes completely or most of the way during the hold maneuvers (Plate 1.7). The scope is further withdrawn until the UVJ closes two thirds of the way. The patient is asked to 'strain down' and 'cough' and the urethroscope is moved to keep the lumen in the visual field. This provides a subjective evaluation of UVJ mobility as the normal UVJ moves minimally or closes with these commands[6] (Fig. 3.1). The urethral hypermobility typical of genuine stress incontinence, causes the UVJ to descend in response to cough and Valsalva maneuver.

A patient who is able to void with the urethroscope in position will have complete relaxation and opening of the urethra (Plate 1.8), followed by smooth closure as voiding ceases.[7]

COMPLETION OF URETHROSCOPIC EXAMINATION

The urethroscopic examination is completed with the bladder full, brisk fluid flow maintained, and compression of the UVJ with the vaginal finger (Fig. 3.2), so as to distend the urethral lumen. The urethral mucosa is pink throughout, with a slightly reddish tinge. Periurethral gland openings are located posteriorly in the distal two thirds of the urethra (Plate 1.9). Inflamed glands may contain expressible fluid or pus when massaged by a finger, or the area may be intensely tender to touch.

A.

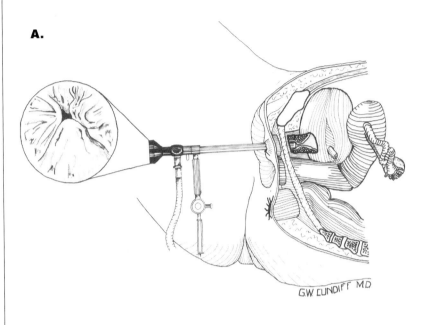

G.W. CUNDIFF M.D.

B.

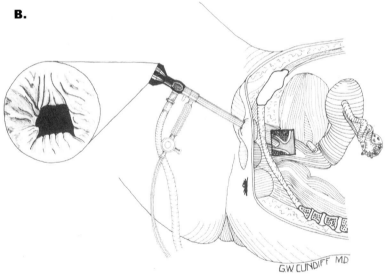

G.W. CUNDIFF M.D.

Fig. 3.1 Demonstrating urethral hypermobility. **a.** The urethroscope is withdrawn to allow the urethra to close by two thirds. **b.** The patient is asked to cough, causing the UVJ to descend and open. Downward deflection of the scope is required to maintain the view of the UVJ

EVALUATION OF THE VESICAL MUCOSA

The cystoscope, preferably the 17F sheath with 30° or 70° lens, is lubricated with 2% xylocaine jelly and inserted into the distal urethra with a 20–30° upward angulation toward the umbilicus.[8] An obturator is not necessary in the female patient. The closed portion of the distal sheath (see Chapter 2) is kept in contact with the posterior aspect of the urethra as the instrument is passed into the bladder. The dome or superior aspect of the bladder is identified by the presence of the air bubble (Plate 1.10). The cystoscope is angled to view each hour

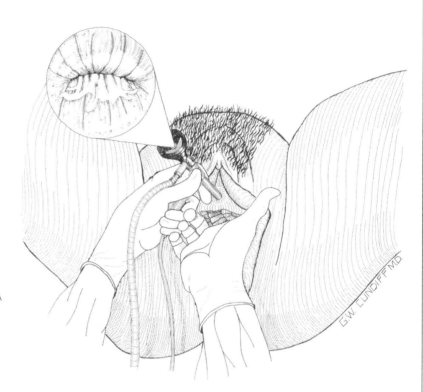

Fig. 3.2 Milking of the urethral glands. A vaginal finger obstructs the proximal urethra, and gentle massage of the urethra against the scope milks exudate from glands and diverticular openings, which helps to localize the ostia

of an imaginary clock as the scope is inserted and withdrawn under direct vision (Figure 3.3). The scope must be close to the bladder wall to allow for greatest illumination, although modern cameras are sensitive to even a small amount of light. A steady slow flow of fluid is maintained, and the bladder is filled close to capacity for best viewing results. The trigone area is examined last, and a vaginal

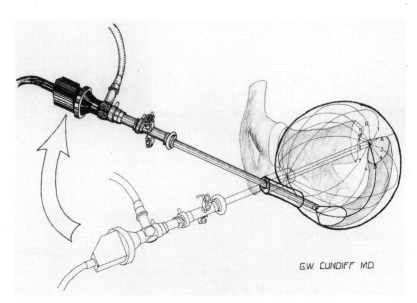

Fig. 3.3 Cystoscopic evaluation of the bladder. The entire bladder cavity is assessed by making 12 sweeps from the bladder dome to the UVJ. The five o'clock sweep is shown. Note that the camera remains upright, while the cystoscope is turned so that the angled view is directed to 5 o'clock

finger may be required to lift the bladder base into view in cases of prolapse where the bladder can be difficult to visualize fully (see Chapter 5). The bladder is filled continually during these observations and note is made of first sensation (normal 50–150 ml), fullness at 250–400 ml, and maximum capacity of 350–550 ml.[9]

CYSTOSCOPIC APPEARANCE OF NORMAL VESICAL ANATOMY

The mucosa is examined for color, vascular appearance, abnormal lesions, and trabeculations. The bladder wall is whitish to pink, with numerous vessels coursing through the tissue (Plate 1.11). At the bladder base is the trigone, an area bounded by the interureteric ridge superiorly, and laterally by the ureteral bars and openings (Plate 1.12). The apex of the trigone is the vesical neck or bladder outlet, also called the UVJ. The trigonal area remains smooth in appearance, and the bladder mucosa is flat when the bladder is filled, but wrinkled when the bladder contains a lesser volume.[8] The trigone almost always appears inflamed, especially near the bladder neck, and a smooth white covering of squamous metaplasia (Plates 1.13 and 1.14) is usually distributed over the trigone area near the interureteric ridge and ureteral bars. Metaplasia does not represent an inflammatory process but may be a developmental migration of vaginal epithelium, or metaplasia of the trigonal mucosa.

Ureteral openings have many shapes and sizes, and should actively spurt urine every few minutes (Plates 1.15–1.17). Each orifice should be observed until efflux of urine is seen. This is preceded by contraction of the ureteral musculature on the lateral ureteric ridge, and then the obvious opening of the ureter occurs. If the cervix and uterus are *in situ*, there will be a smooth posterior cushion of tissue pushing up into the bladder wall with recesses or vestibules on either side (Plate 1.18).

NONPATHOLOGIC ABNORMALITIES

Urethral septa are not common and are usually asymptomatic (Plates 2.1 and 2.2). Fronds may be present at the UVJ (Plates 2.3 and 2.4), and polyps occur at the UVJ (Plate 2.5) or in the urethra (Plate 2.6). Vesical and ureteral variations may be anatomic or functional abnormalities. Accessory ureteral orifices are one anatomic abnormality indicative of renal collecting anomalies. Many enter the bladder slightly superiorly to the trigone in close proximity to the normal ureteral orifice (Plates 2.7 and 2.8). Ureteroceles are due to laxity of the distal ureteral lumen with herniation into the vesical cavity just before efflux (Plate 2.9).

Trabeculations are common findings, especially in the elderly, and the smooth ridges become more evident as the bladder is filled to capacity. They appear as interlaced cords of different diameters and intervening sacculations (Plates 2.10–2.12). Their significance is not certain, but may represent hypertrophied detrusor muscle associated with detrusor instability and functional or anatomic outlet obstruction. A bladder diverticulum is an enlarged sacculation in the bladder wall (Plate 2.13). The interior of the diverticulum has been reported as the site of neoplasm in approximately 7% of cases.[10]

Bladder wall scarring usually occurs after bladder injury with penetration of the wall, but, once healing is complete, symptoms are unusual (Plates 2.14 and 2.15). Fistulas may leave tell-tale signs of previous problems (Plate 2.16).

COMPLICATIONS OF CYSTOURETHROSCOPY (Table 3.2)

Infection is the most significant cause of morbidity after cystoscopy, although the actual rate of procedural infection is not well known. The rate of bacteriuria has been cited as 2.8–16.6%.[11–14] The concern regarding potential morbidity has prompted physicians to use prophylactic antibiotics, most commonly nitrofurantoin for 1–3 days. A recent report of a randomized double-blind placebo-controlled evaluation of nitrofurantoin prophylaxis for combined urodynamics and cystourethroscopy failed to show any benefit in decreasing postinstrumentation bacteriuria or urinary tract infection.[14] While this was the largest prospective study to date, it had a power of only 33%, and consequently the benefit of antibiotic prophylaxis remains debatable. Certainly, pyelonephritis is an uncommon complication, but must be managed promptly with appropriate antibiotics.

The most frequent complication is urgency or burning with urination, secondary to irritation of the bladder wall and urethra. Patients

Table 3.2 Complications of cystourethroscopy

Painful urination
Hematuria
Urinary tract infection
Difficulty voiding
Bladder spasms
Urethral spasms
Exacerbation of urinary tract symptoms
Reaction to prophylactic antibiotics

may experience short-term hematuria. Patients with preoperative irritative voiding symptoms may have a marked exacerbation of these symptoms. The inability to void or worsening of incontinence is an unlikely consequence of the procedure. Phenazopyridine is administered for urinary discomfort for two or three doses.

REFERENCES

1. Carter HB. Instrumentation and Endoscopy. In Walsh PC, Retik AB, Stamey TA, Vaughan ED (eds) *Campbell's Urology*, 6th edn. Philadelphia: WB Saunders, 1992: 335–7.
2. Robertson JR. Dynamic urethroscopy. In Ostergard DR, Bent AE (eds) *Urogynecology and Urodynamics: Theory and Practice*, 4th edn. Baltimore: Williams and Wilkins, 1996: 165–72.
3. Schonebeck J. Normal anatomy. In *Atlas of Cystoscopy*. Orlando: Grune and Stratton, 1985: 19–28.
4. Hinman F Jr. Bladder and ureterovesical junction: structure and function. In *Atlas of Urological Anatomy*. Philadelphia: WB Saunders, 1993: 331–9.
5. Bagley DH, Huffman JL, Lyon ES. Normal anatomy of the urethra, prostate, and bladder. In Bagley DH, Huffman JL, Lyon ES (eds) *Urologic Endoscopy: A Manual and Atlas*. Boston: Little, Brown, 1985: 3–11.
6. Bent AE, Ostergard DR. Urethrocystoscopy. In Sanfilippo JS, Levine RL (eds) *Operative Gynecologic Endoscopy*. New York: Springer, 1989: 272–80.
7. O'Donnell P. Endoscopy. In Raz S (ed.) *Female Urology*. Philadelphia: WB Saunders, 1983: 51–68.
8. Bagley DH, Huffman JL, Lyon ES. Cystourethroscopy. In Bagley DH, Huffman JL, Lyon ES (eds) *Urologic Endoscopy: A Manual and Atlas*. Boston: Little, Brown, 1985: 77–97.
9. Cundiff GW, Bent AE. Cystoscopy for the urogynecologist. In Ostergard DR, Bent AE (eds) *Urogynecology and Urodynamics: Theory and Practice*. 4th edn. Baltimore: Williams and Wilkins, 1996: 173–86.
10. Kelalis PP, McLean P. The treatment of diverticulum of the bladder. *J Urol* 1967; **98**: 349–52.
11. Manson AL. Is antibiotic prophylaxis indicated after outpatient cystoscopy? *J Urol* 1988; **140**: 316–17.
12. Richards B, Bastable JRG. Bacteriuria after outpatient cystoscopy. *Br J Urol* 1977; **49**: 561–4.
13. Hares MM. A double-blinded trial of half-strength Polybactrin soluble GU bladder irrigations in cystoscopy. *Br J Urol* 1981; **53**: 62–67.
14. Cundiff GW, McLennan MT, Bent AE. Double-blinded randomized evaluation of nitrofurantoin prophylaxis for combined urodynamics and cystourethroscopy. Annual meeting of the American Urogynecologic Society, September 24–28, 1997, Tucson, Arizona (abstract).

CHAPTER 4

Irritative voiding symptoms

Alfred E. Bent

DIFFERENTIAL DIAGNOSIS AND INDICATIONS FOR ENDOSCOPY

The differential diagnosis for irritative voiding symptoms is extensive and includes many conditions that are nebulous and therefore hard to describe in precise terms. The following disorders should be considered: acute cystitis, chronic cystitis, trigonitis, radiation cystitis, urethral syndrome, urethral diverticula, urethritis, and interstitial cystitis. Other conditions that may cause similar symptoms but are not considered in this chapter include detrusor instability, sensory urge incontinence, bladder or ureteral stones, bladder tumor, partial urinary retention, and moderate or severe pelvic organ prolapse (Table 4.1).

Endoscopy is indicated when the presenting symptoms strongly suggest a diagnosis of urethral diverticulum, interstitial cystitis, stone disease, or tumor. Most other conditions can be treated after taking a history, physical examination, and microscopic examination of the urine. If response to therapy does not occur, endoscopy should be considered as part of the evaluation process. It would be inappropriate to perform endoscopy knowingly in the presence of infection of the lower or upper urinary tract.

URETHRITIS

Acute urethritis may be most frequently caused by *Chlamydia trachomatis*, *Neisseria gonorrhea*, *Mycoplasma hominis*, and *Ureaplasma urealyiticum* (Plate 3.1). Other bacteria common in lower urinary tract infections have been implicated in acute urethritis, but, when cultured, very low colony counts may be obtained. Other causes of acute urethritis include trauma, instrumentation (catheters), bubble baths, perineal sprays, sexual intercourse, and tampon insertion. The

Table 4.1 Differential diagnosis of irritative voiding symptoms

Urethritis
Urethral syndrome
Urethral diverticulum
Acute cystitis
Chronic cystitis
Trigonitis
Radiation cystitis
Urge incontinence
Bladder or ureteral stones
Bladder tumor
Urinary retention
Pelvic organ prolapse

urethral findings at urethroscopy are nonspecific and include inflammatory urethral mucosa, bleeding areas, superficial ulceration of urethral mucosa (trauma), and exudate on the mucosal surface.

URETHRAL SYNDROME

Urethral syndrome is a chronic (6 months or greater) irritative condition of the lower urinary tract, specifically the urethra, associated especially with urgency and frequency, in the absence of obvious bladder or urethral abnormalities or significant bacterial growth in the urine.[1] The findings at urethroscopy may include redness of urethral mucosa (Plate 3.2), debris or exudate expressed from posterior periurethral glands (Plate 3.3), and inflammatory fronds or polyps in the proximal urethra or urethrovesical junction (Plates 2.3 and 2.4), although these findings are not diagnostic as they are found in asymptomatic patients. Cystoscopy may reveal an associated severe form of trigonitis. Quite commonly there are no specific findings at urethroscopy, and a normal exam is reported. Treatment is then based on symptom relief and reversal of the urge–void cycle through a combination of medication, bladder retraining, and education.

ATROPHIC URETHRITIS

Atrophic urethritis may be acute or chronic, and results from lack of estrogen support. There are several studies documenting estrogen receptors in the urethra, and the use of oral or topical estrogen to reverse symptoms of urgency and frequency. The urethral mucosa in the hypoestrogenic patient is pale, and may be stenotic or friable (Plate 3.4).

URETHRAL DIVERTICULA

Urethral diverticula occur in 1–3% of women, and are located along the posterior–lateral wall of the urethra as single or multiple outpouchings. The classic symptom of postvoid dribbling almost never occurs at presentation, but frequently reported symptoms include recurrent urinary tract infection (UTI), urinary incontinence, and a painful swelling in the anterior vagina, with or without expression of pus by massaging the urethra.[2] Chronic pelvic pain may be the only symptom. Over half of the diverticular openings are at the midurethra, with a number more proximal, and some more distal.[3] The most common radiologic procedures for diagnosis are voiding cystourethrography and positive pressure urethrography using a Tratner or Davis triple-lumen catheter. The urethroscopic diagnosis may be as accurate as the radiographic techniques, provided the bladder is filled and the bladder neck or proximal urethra is occluded by the vaginal finger. A steady flow of fluid is maintained into the urethra as the scope is withdrawn and urethra massaged by the vaginal finger pressing upward from below. This is one instance when carbon dioxide gas infusion is preferable to water or saline for urethroscopy (Plates 3.5–3.8).

ACUTE CYSTITIS

Acute cystitis is an acute inflammation of the bladder, usually with symptoms of urinary frequency, urgency, and dysuria.[4] The vast majority of acute inflammations of the bladder are caused by coliform bacteria which are readily treated after microscopic, dipstick, or culture confirmation. Less commonly, the offenders can be viral, fungal, or protozoal agents. Nonbiologic agents causing cystitis include physical trauma (catheterization or instrumentation), radiation, and chemotherapeutic agents.[5] It is unusual to perform endoscopy in the acute phase of inflammation, and more often it occurs by chance when performed as part of evaluation of the lower urinary tract for persisting irritative symptoms, hematuria, or incontinence. Endoscopic findings include a relatively normal appearing bladder or hypervascularity in mild inflammations (Plates 3.9 and 3.10), dulling of the sharp vascular pattern due to mucosal edema (Plate 3.11), soft pink to red inflamed areas with indefinite borders (Plate 3.12), numerous small petechiae on the bladder surface (Plate 3.13), more obvious red discoid or patchy hemorrhagic areas (Plates 3.14), or confluent mucosal hemorrhages and frank hemorrhage in severe cases (Plates 3.15 and 3.16). The exudate can be sufficiently varied to look like tumor material, and a combination of biopsy, urine culture, and antibacterial treatment usually effects a dramatic change in the bladder appearance within 2 weeks. Catheter or polypoid cystitis is associated mostly with indwelling catheters and occurs along the posterior wall and dome of the bladder (Plate 3.17). It is characterized by inflammatory polyps which are edematous and may bleed easily.[6]

CHRONIC CYSTITIS

Chronic cystitis by definition means that an irritative condition has been present for more than 3–6 months. Asymptomatic bacteriuria may be present for many months but is not associated with symptoms, and usually has minimal impact on changes to be observed on the bladder mucosa. A chronic low-grade bladder infection will usually produce some mild irritative voiding symptoms and endoscopy may reveal inflammatory patches in the mucosa, or areas of discrete pink or red macules in part or all of the bladder (Plate 3.18). A virulent bacterial acute inflammation is very unlikely to become chronic, because the severity of symptoms would have necessitated therapy.

TRIGONITIS

Trigonitis is an irritated appearing trigone, with red petechial areas over the trigone as it rises from the urethrovesical junction, and usually a white membranous epithelium reaching in tongue-like fashion toward the interureteric ridge. Another description is confluent areas of pearly-gray granular epithelium with irregular margins. The membrane is due to stratified squamous epithelium, and histologic evaluation reveals squamous metaplasia, usually referred to as metaplasia. The term pseudomembranous trigonitis has been used in the past, but is best avoided in this condition. The significance of the condition is uncertain, and, while some think it can cause irritative voiding symptoms, others see it as a normal variant (Plates 3.19 and 3.20).

RADIATION CYSTITIS

Many types of chronic cystitis are caused by specific agents that have characteristic findings. Acute radiation changes are uncommon in current practice. The range of findings is from mucosal hyperemia, to superficial ulcerations, to severe irritability of the bladder. Symptoms include urinary frequency, urgency, and possibly hematuria. Late changes from radiation therapy are much more common as a result of fibrosis and thickening in the walls of blood vessels as well as hyalinization of connective tissue. A loss of vascularity in the submucosa causes a paleness in the bladder mucosa, with loss of vascular pattern[6,7] (Plate 3.21). Symptoms include irritative symptoms or severe urgency due to a contracted bladder. Uncommon causes of chronic cystitis not discussed further include tuberculosis, schistosomal cystitis, and eosinophilic cystitis.

INTERSTITIAL CYSTITIS

Interstitial cystitis is a chronic inflammatory disorder of full-thickness bladder wall. It is characterized by progressive symptoms of urinary frequency, urgency, suprapubic pain, and nocturia. Typically the pain worsens as the bladder fills, and lessens with voiding.[8]

Patients do not generally report urinary incontinence. Attempts at cystoscopic examination or cystometry under local anesthesia are very difficult owing to the small bladder capacity which in severe cases may be as low as 50 ml. Endoscopy performed under general anesthesia is usually more successful in making a diagnosis, and should consist of two phases. Initial examination includes an inspection of the bladder wall and obtaining urine for culture and cytology. The second phase of examination consists of hydrodistension with the infusion bag at 80–100 cm above the symphysis, and compressing the female urethra during filling to prevent leakage. After refill of the bladder, glomerulations (petechiae) will appear throughout the bladder lining, mostly in the dome, posterior, and lateral walls. More severe cases will show linear fissures in the mucosa, as well as splotchy hemorrhages.[7] The finding of Hunner's ulcer is extremely uncommon, and less than 8% of patients have this finding. A Hunner ulcer is characterized by central ulceration with stellate scars radiating from it. Patients with early forms of interstitial cystitis may not have positive findings at cystoscopy. Biopsy is performed only to rule out carcinoma *in situ*, and is not diagnostic for interstitial cystitis (Plates 3.22–3.26).

REFERENCES

1. Scotti RJ, Ostergard DR. Urethral syndrome. In Ostergard DR, Bent AE (eds) *Urogynecology and Urodynamics: Theory and Practice*. Baltimore: Williams and Wilkins, 1996: 339–59.
2. Petersen RO. Urethra. In *Urologic Pathology*. Philadelphia: JB Lippincott, 1986: 417–52.
3. Robertson JR. Urethral diverticula. In Ostergard DR, Bent AE (eds) *Urogynecology and Urodynamics: Theory and Practice*. Baltimore: Williams and Wilkins, 1996: 361–70.
4. Karram MM. Lower urinary tract infection. In Ostergard DR, Bent AE (eds) *Urogynecology and Urodynamics: Theory and Practice*. Baltimore: Williams and Wilkins, 1996: Chapter 28, 387–408.
5. Petersen RO. Urinary bladder. In *Urologic Pathology*. Philadelphia: JB Lippincott, 1986: 279–416.
6. Bagley DH, Huffman JL, Lyon ES. Abnormal bladder. In Bagley DH, Huffman JL, Lyon ES (eds) *Urologic Endoscopy: A Manual and Atlas*. Boston: Little, Brown, 1985: 41–58.
7. O'Donnell P. Water endoscopy. In *Female Urology*. Philadelphia: WB Saunders, 1983: 51–68.
8. Parsons CL. Interstitial cystitis. In Ostergard DR, Bent AE (eds) *Urogynecology and Urodynamics: Theory and Practice*. Baltimore: Williams and Wilkins, 1996: 409–25.

CHAPTER 5

Urinary incontinence

Geoffrey W. Cundiff

DIFFERENTIAL DIAGNOSIS AND INDICATIONS FOR ENDOSCOPY

Dynamic urethroscopy was proposed as a comprehensive method of evaluating lower urinary tract dysfunction nearly thirty years ago[1] and continues to provide important diagnostic information in the evaluation of incontinence in women. There is general agreement that cystoscopy is indicated for patients complaining of irritative symptoms, hematuria, persistent incontinence, or voiding dysfunction following incontinence surgery (Table 5.1). There is less agreement about the role of cystoscopy in the baseline evaluation of the patient with urinary incontinence and there are relatively few analyses to define its role in this capacity.

The refinement of urodynamic evaluation over the past 3 decades has demonstrated the superiority of this method for diagnosing the common etiologies of urinary incontinence such as genuine stress incontinence and detrusor instability.[2,3] However, while urodynamics excels at providing an objective assessment of lower urinary tract function, it provides relatively little information about anatomy. Urethrocystoscopy contributes an anatomic assessment of the urethra and bladder, and allows discovery of benign and malignant mucosal lesions that would remain undiagnosed by urodynamics alone.

Mucosal lesions

The value of urethrocystoscopy as an adjuvant to urodynamics is illustrated in a report by Cundiff and Bent.[4] In this study of women undergoing combined urodynamics and urethrocystoscopy, urethrocystoscopy was considered important to 19% of the final diagnoses. Specifically, it provided new information in patients with anatomic abnormalities including malignant and premalignant intravesical lesions. These conditions are discussed in Chapter 6.

Table 5.1 Indications for cystourethroscopy during incontinence evaluation: historical indicators

Hematuria
Irritative voiding symptoms
Risk factors for bladder cancer
Recurrent incontinence
Posttraumatic incontinence
Puerperal incontinence
Posthysterectomy incontinence
Risk factors for intrinsic sphincteric deficiency
Voiding dysfunction
Postvoid dribbling

Anatomic abnormalities

Other anatomic abnormalities might be suspected based on history or urodynamics but require an anatomic assessment for confirmation. These include urethral diverticula (see Chapter 7), urinary–vaginal fistulas (see Chapter 8), and intravesical foreign bodies causing detrusor instability (see Chapter 6). For example, a diverticulum can be suspected based on a history of recurrent urinary tract infections, postvoid dribbling, or pelvic pain. In such a patient a biphasic urethral pressure profile is virtually diagnostic of a urethral diverticulum, yet Leach and Bavendam[5] noted this finding in only 28% of patients with a urethral diverticulum. This contrasts with the reported diagnostic accuracy of urethrocystoscopy of 84–90%.[6,7] Urethrocystoscopy not only confirms the diverticulum but also provides important information about the size and location of the ostia, as well as the presence of multiple diverticula.

The ability of cystourethroscopy to define the location, size, and surrounding anatomic relationships pertains for urinary–vaginal fistula as well, and both Massee et al.[8] and Symmonds[9] consider it the simplest method of evaluating urinary tract fistula.

Intrinsic sphincteric deficiency

Urethrocystoscopy may also have a role in the diagnosis of intrinsic sphincteric deficiency. The Agency for Health Care Policy and Research coined the term intrinsic sphincteric deficiency, and defined it conceptually as a condition in which 'the urethral sphincter is unable to coapt and generate enough resistance to retain urine in the bladder'.[10] Unfortunately, the clinical criteria for intrinsic sphincteric deficiency have not been defined. Some have used a single urodynamic parameter. In the absence of validated standard criteria for diagnosing intrinsic sphincteric deficiency, an approach that combines historical risk factors with urodynamic evidence of poor urethral resistance and an anatomic evaluation of urethral coaptation seems to be warranted. Cystourethroscopy is perhaps the simplest approach to achieve an anatomic evaluation of the urethrovesical junction (UVJ). In comparing low maximum urethral closure pressure (MUCP) to a composite diagnostic criteria based on history, urodynamics, and endoscopic appearance of the UVJ, Cundiff and Bent reported that low MUCP (20 cm of H_2O) had a sensitivity of 20% and a positive predictive value of 40% for diagnosing intrinsic sphincteric deficiency.[4]

The anatomic evaluation provided by cystourethroscopy can also be achieved using radiological techniques, including fluoroscopy and transrectal or perineal ultrasonography.[11–14] When properly performed, urethroscopy provides an equivalent anatomic evaluation of the UVJ to that provided by video urodynamics, but the cost of providing basic urethrocystoscopy is considerably lower. Moreover, urethrocystoscopy provides an evaluation of the lower urinary tract mucosa not achieved by radiographic modalities.

CYSTOURETHROSCOPIC TECHNIQUES

A complete endoscopic evaluation for urinary incontinence requires evaluation of both the bladder and urethra. The technique of diagnostic cystourethroscopy is outlined in detail in Chapter 3. There are several techniques that augment diagnostic urethroscopy and cystoscopy in the evaluation of urinary incontinence, including dynamic urethroscopy. Dynamic urethroscopy is discussed in Chapter 3, and endoscopic techniques to evaluate urogenital fistulas are discussed in Chapter 8.

URETHROCYSTOSCOPIC FINDINGS IN INCONTINENT WOMEN

Genuine stress incontinence

The poor support of the UVJ present in genuine stress incontinence due to urethral hypermobility permits descent and may cause gaping of the UVJ, often referred to as 'funneling'. Urethroscopic findings typical of the patient with intrinsic sphincteric deficiency include poor coaptation (Plate 4.1), often with a short rigid immobile urethra (Plate 4.2). In severe cases, the UVJ is unresponsive to commands and the lumen is visualized in its entirety from meatus to UVJ (Plate 4.3).

Detrusor instability

Detrusor instability is suspected if there is uncontrollable urethral opening during filling. Trabeculations are also a common finding in women with detrusor instability, although they are not diagnostic of this condition (Plates 2.10–2.12).

Other causes of incontinence

Urinary incontinence that is not associated with urgency or stress may be due to urethral diverticula (Plates 3.5–3.8), vesicovaginal fistula (Plates 6.1–6.3) or urethrovaginal fistula (Plates 6.4 and 6.5). These topics are addressed in Chapters 7 and 8 respectively. Intravesical foreign bodies (Plates 4.4–4.10) may present with hematuria (see Chapter 6) or as urge incontinence, as the mucosal irritation can cause detrusor instability. Cystourethroscopy can provide valuable information in making these diagnoses.

Pelvic organ prolapse

A subjective prediction of the architectural support of the bladder base can be made from the cystoscopic view of the base and the position of bladder base structures. This is best accomplished with the angled scope oriented to view the bladder base and positioned at the UVJ to provide a panoramic view.

The bladder rests on the trapezoid-shaped pubocervical fascia which is stretched between the arcus tendineus fasciae pelvis on either side. The arcus tendineus fasciae pelvis is the condensation of the pubocervical fascia as it intercepts the fascia of the obturator internus muscle. They run from the posterior aspect of the symphysis pubis to the ischial spine. Superiorly the pubocervical fascia is contiguous with the cervix, which often protrudes into the bladder base creating recesses or vestibules laterally.

In patients with paravaginal defects, there is an exaggeration of these recesses as the lateral support of the bladder is compromised (Plate 4.11). This loss of lateral support also changes the position of the ureteral orifices, which sag medially and may be seen in near apposition (kissing ureters) in women with bilateral paravaginal defects (Plate 4.12).

A midline defect in the pubocervical fascia is visualized as a drop off of the trigone and bladder base which may require a vaginal finger to visualize fully the mucosa of the base (Plate 4.13).

A superior defect in the pubocervical fascia is seen as a sagging of the bladder dome with support of the trigone. The lateral position of the ureteral orifices tends to be preserved in this support defect. Combinations of paravaginal and midline defects can also be deduced from combinations of these findings (Plate 4.14).

CONCLUSION

Urethrocystoscopy is a valuable technique in the evaluation of urinary incontinence in women. While less sensitive and specific than multichannel urodynamics for the most common etiologies of incontinence, it provides an anatomic assessment of the urethra and bladder that is not accomplished with urodynamics alone. This allows for the discovery of benign and malignant mucosal lesions. Additionally, cystourethroscopy facilitates the diagnosis of intrinsic sphincteric deficiency and provides a subjective assessment of the support of the urethrovesical junction and bladder base.

REFERENCES

1. Robertson JR. Air cystoscopy. *Obstet Gynecol* 1968; **32**: 328–30.
2. Sand PK, Hill RC, Ostergard DR. Supine urethroscopic and standing cystometry as screening methods for detection of detrusor instability. *Obstet Gynecol* 1987; **70**: 57–60.
3. Scotti RJ, Ostergard DR, Guillaume AA, Kohatsu KE. Predictive value of urethroscopy as compared to urodynamics in the diagnosis of genuine stress incontinence. *J Reprod Med* 1990; **35**: 772–6.
4. Cundiff GW, Bent AE. The contribution of urethrocystoscopy to a combined urodynamic and urethrocystoscopic evaluation of urinary incontinence in women. *Int J Urogynecol* 1996; **7**: 307–11.
5. Leach GE, Bavendam TG. Female urethral diverticula. *Urology* 1987; **30**: 407–15.
6. Robertson JR. Urethral diverticula. In Ostergard DR, Bent AE (eds) *Urogynecology and Urodynamics: Theory and Practice*, 3rd edn. Baltimore: Williams and Wilkins, 1991: 283–91.
7. Drutz HP. Urethral diverticula. *Obstet Gynecol Clin North Am* 1989; **16**: 923–9.
8. Massee JS, Welch JS, Pratt JH, Symmonds RE. Management of urinary–vaginal fistula. *JAMA* 1964; **190**: 124–8.
9. Symmonds RE. Incontinence: vesical and urethral fistulas. *Clin Obstet Gynecol* 1984; **27**: 499–514.
10. Urinary Incontinence Guideline Panel. *Urinary Incontinence in Adults: Clinical Practical Guidelines*. AHCPR Pub. No. 92-0038. Rockville, MD: Agency for Health Care Policy and Research, Public Health Service, US Department of Health and Human Services, March 1992.
11. Bergman A, McKenzie CJ, Richmond J, Ballard CA, Platt LD. Transrectal ultrasound versus cystography in the evaluation of anatomical stress urinary incontinence. *Br J Urol* 1988; **62**: 228–34.
12. Chang HC, Chang SC, Kuo HC, Tsai TC. Transrectal sonographic cystourethrography: studies in stress urinary incontinence. *Urology* 1990; **36**: 488–92.
13. Gordon D, Pearce M, Norton P, Stanton S. Comparison of ultrasound and lateral chain urethrocystography in the determination of bladder neck descent. *Am J Obstet Gynecol* 1989; **160**: 182–5.
14. Weil EHK, van Waalaijk van Doorn ESC, Heesakkers JPFA, Meguid T, Janknegt RA. Transvaginal ultrasonogrpahy: a study with healthy volunteers and women with genuine stress incontinence. *Eur Urol* 1993; **24**: 226–30.

CHAPTER 6

Hematuria

Alfred E. Bent

DIFFERENTIAL DIAGNOSIS AND INDICATIONS FOR ENDOSCOPY

Hematuria is the excretion of abnormal quantities of red blood cells in the urine, which may present as gross or microscopic hematuria. Several types of dipstick tests have been used for screening purposes, but approximately 10% of patients with microscopic hematuria are missed. The best method of detection is microscopic examination of a first-voided morning urine specimen, which is centrifuged for 3–5 minutes. The upper limit of normal is three erythrocytes per high-power field, although 3% of normal individuals excrete more than that amount.[1]

The differential diagnosis for hematuria is extensive (Table 6.1), but falls into conditions that are primarily of renal (glomerular and nonglomerular) or postrenal origin. The kinds of conditions for which endoscopy is helpful in diagnosis are bladder cancer and other neoplastic lesions of the bladder wall, chronic cystitis, foreign body, urolithiasis, recurrent cystitis, interstitial cystitis, and urethral lesions such as polyps, acute inflammation, and cancer. The medical conditions may require assessment for proteinuria, morphologic assessment of the urinary red cells, urine chemistries for hypercalciuria or hyperuricosuria, urine culture, renal function studies, screening blood chemistries, complete blood count with peripheral smear, coagulation profile, erythrocyte sedimentation rate, and kidney biopsy. Renal ultrasonography and/or intravenous urography are important for both renal and postrenal conditions, with

---

Table 6.1 Differential diagnosis of hematuria

Renal
  Glomerular
  Nonglomerular

Bladder
  Cancer of the bladder
  Other neoplastic conditions of the bladder wall
  Acute cystitis or other inflammation
  Chronic cystitis
  Interstitial cystitis
  Foreign body
  Urolithiasis
  Trauma

Urethra
  Polyps
  Acute inflammation
  Cancer
  Prolapse
  Caruncle
  Trauma

---

particular importance in cancer of the kidney and in urolithiasis. Urine cytology is an important adjunct in the detection of bladder cancer. Patients referred with gross hematuria in the absence of infection should have renal ultrasonography or intravenous urography, urine for cytology, and cystourethroscopy. Patients with microscopic hematuria and a sterile urine, with a normal medical work-up, require the same evaluation.

BENIGN AND MALIGNANT CONDITIONS OF THE URETHRA

A urethral caruncle is an inflammatory lesion on the posterior aspect of the distal urethra clinically associated with pain and bleeding. The appearance is that of a very red area of mucosal surface spilling out of the distal posterior urethra, measuring 5–10 mm in size (Plate 5.1). Urethral prolapse is a circumferential red mucosal eversion at the urethral meatus. It is not usually tender, but often bleeds. It may occur in the very young, as well as in the postmenopausal woman. It generally responds well to topical estrogen therapy (Plate 5.2).

Polypoid urethritis is a proliferative tissue reaction to chronic inflammation as a result of an indwelling catheter. The exophytic polypoid projections are inflamed and may have superficial ulceration. Other benign-appearing polyps occur in the urethra and may give rise to bleeding especially if traumatized in any manner (Plate 5.3).

Cancer of the urethra is uncommon, but is the only urinary tract tumor in which the frequency is greater in women than men. The histologic types are squamous, transitional, adenocarcinoma, and malignant melanoma in order of decreasing frequency. Most patients present with urethral bleeding or dysuria, but most tumors have already spread to adjacent tissues at diagnosis, and prognosis is poor.[2]

FOREIGN BODIES

Bladder calculi may form as a result of urinary stasis and infected urine, or around a foreign body. Most foreign bodies arrive in the bladder by iatrogenic means, generally at the time of bladder neck suspension procedures. The types of foreign materials include sutures, buttresses from needle suspension procedures, and sling materials. Secondary to the foreign body, there may be an inflammatory reaction in the bladder (Plates 4.7 and 5.4).

BENIGN NEOPLASTIC LESIONS OF THE BLADDER

Cystitis cystica are islands of benign-appearing urothelium situated in the submucosa resulting from inward proliferation of basal cells (Plates 5.5 and 5.6). The centers have undergone eosinophilic liquefaction. The color reflects the liquid center and may vary from clear, to yellow/brown, to black.[3] The lesions may also arise from subepithelial islands of transitional cells, known as Brunn's nests.[4] They occur in 60% of normal bladders at autopsy.[5] The lesions are clear, 2–5 mm in size, and appear as small nodules mostly over the trigone and bladder base, but sometimes on the lateral walls. While older literature assumes the etiology as chronic irritation, the lesions may be a normal proliferative variant of urothelium.

Cystitis glandularis is similar to cystitis cystica except the transitional cells have undergone glandular hyperplasia, creating a structure with a goblet cell lining. The cysts are macroscopically larger and more irregular,[3] suggesting a premalignant change, although this is very rare. Other appearances are those of a papillary or cystic red lesion (Plate 5.7).

Endometriosis occurs in the bladder more frequently than other locations in the urinary tract, although it is not common. It is usually observed in patients in the fourth decade, who may present with pelvic pain, pressure, urinary urgency, frequency, and hematuria in one fourth of cases. The lesion may be suspected at cystoscopy only if it is impinging on lamina propria, or of course through to mucosal surface. Most lesions are in the muscle or subserosa. Biopsy has not been helpful in diagnosis in the past, but the classic features of endometrial glands, investing stroma, and histologic evidence of past hemorrhage are characteristic (Plate 5.8).

Transitional cell papilloma is a papillary neoplasm of the urothelial mucosal epithelium (with a well defined vascular stalk), which on histology shows normal epithelium. Usually the lesions are single, 2–5 cm in diameter, and represent 2–3% of bladder tumors (Plate 5.9). The problem with this diagnosis is that recurrence is frequent, and the risk of malignant change cannot be overlooked. Therefore, the patient should be followed as if a malignant lesion had been found, and have regular examinations.

MALIGNANT NEOPLASTIC LESIONS OF THE BLADDER

Epithelial neoplasms constitute over 98% of bladder tumors, with most being transitional cell carcinoma. The types of tumor include transitional cell carcinoma, squamous cell carcinoma (verrucous type) making up only 5% of cancers, and adenocarcinoma (mucinous, signet ring, and clear cell carcinomas), comprising only 2% of tumors. Bladder cancer is the eighth most common cancer in women, accounting for 4% of cancers. There are over 12 000 cases per year in women in the United States, and the tumor is three times more common in men.[4,5]

Transitional cell carcinoma *in situ* is characterized by flat (nonpapillary) urothelial cell proliferation with full-thickness dysplasia, but no invasion of the basement membrane. However, many of these lesions can progress to malignant change, or may be found in association with invasive carcinoma. Therefore close follow-up is recommended.

Transitional cell carcinoma is associated with hematuria in 70–95% of cases, and with dysuria in 20%. The neoplasm measures from a few millimeters to several centimeters, and is most often located at the lateral walls or posterior wall, often just lateral to the ureteral orifices. It is pink in color, papillary, and exophytic. Higher grade lesions may be infiltrating (Plates 5.10–5.13).

Squamous cell carcinoma is an infiltrating and ulcerating lesion, rather than an exophytic papillary mass characteristic of transitional cell carcinoma. Most of these tumors have already invaded bladder wall.

MALIGNANT NEOPLASTIC LESIONS OF SURROUNDING ORGANS

Metastases from other organs account for 5% of tumors of the bladder. The most frequent are malignant melanoma, stomach, breast, and lung. Spread from adjacent organs is more common, especially cervix and uterus (Plate 5.14). Bladder metastases are late occurrences, and most are found at autopsy. Rarely, hematuria is a problem, requiring surgical resection of metastatic tumors to control bleeding.[6]

REFERENCES

1. Schaeffer AJ, Del Greco FD. Other renal diseases of urologic significance. In Walsh PC, Retik AB, Stamey TA, Vaughan ED Jr (eds) *Campbell's Urology*, 6th edn. Philadelphia: WB Saunders, 1992: 2065–81.
2. Petersen RO. Urethra. In *Urologic Pathology*. Philadelphia: JB Lippincott, 1986: 417–52.
3. Schonebeck J. Other bladder changes. In *Atlas of Cystoscopy*. Orlando: Grune and Stratton, 1985: 85–102.
4. Bagley DH, Huffman DL, Lyon ES. Abnormal bladder. In Bagley DH, Huffman DL, Lyon ES (eds) *Urologic Endoscopy: a manual and atlas*. Boston: Little, Brown, 1985: 41–58.
5. Catalona WJ. Urothelial tumors of the urinary tract. In Walsh PC, Retik AB, Stamey

TA, Vaughan ED Jr (eds) *Campbell's Urology*, 6th edn. Philadelphia: WB Saunders, 1992: 1094–1158.

6. Petersen RO. Urinary bladder. In *Urologic Pathology*. Philadelphia: JB Lippincott, 1986: 279–416.

HEMATURIA

CHAPTER 7

Urethral
diverticula

Geoffrey W. Cundiff

DEFINITION

A urethral diverticulum is a circumscribed, fluid-filled out-pouching of the urethral mucous membrane through the urethral muscularis. Hey[1] first reported the successful repair of a urethral diverticulum in 1805. This was considered to be an infrequent malady even into the mid-twentieth century. As recently as 1953 Novack[2] stated, 'This [urethral diverticulum] is a relatively rare condition and no gynecologist will see more than a few in a lifetime.' This viewpoint was supported by the literature as only 17 cases were reported between 1894 and 1954; however, three times this many were reported the following year at Johns Hopkins alone.[3] This increase can be attributed in part to an increase in physician awareness, but was also paralleled with the introduction of new diagnostic modalities. Positive-pressure urethrography, pioneered by Davis and Cain in 1956,[4] was a vast improvement over clinical examination in detecting urethral diverticula. Robertson's introduction of urethroscopy provided yet another easy and reliable technique for diagnosing urethral diverticula.

EPIDEMIOLOGY

Estimations for the prevalence of diverticula in the female urethra range from 1.9% to 4.1%.[5,6] Defining the prevalence of urethral diverticula is complicated by the fact that they may be asymptomatic. Utilizing positive-pressure urethrography in the evaluation of 300 women without urinary complaints, Anderson[6] detected a 3% prevalence in this asymptomatic population. Nevertheless, many women do develop symptoms attributable to urethral diverticula, reflected by a reported 5% prevalence of diverticula in a gynecologic urology clinic population.[7]

The incidence of urethral diverticulum may vary between different races as the condition is reportedly two to six times more common in black women than in white women.[8,9] Typically diverticula are diagnosed between the third and fifth decades.[10] They have been reported in neonates[11] and preadolescent females,[12] although these diverticula may represent congenital malformations and may have a different etiology than those presenting later in life.

ETIOLOGY

Although the etiology of urethral diverticulum has not been clearly determined, multiple etiologies have been proposed. An etiologic classification is presented in Table 7.1. The congenital basis for

Table 7.1 Etiology of urethral diverticula

Congenital
Infection
Trauma
   Instrumentation
   Parturition
   Surgery

diverticula is suggested by their presence in neonates, although this is probably not the etiology for most diverticula. A Gartner duct remnant, a müllerian remnant, 'cell rests,' and faulty union of primal folds have all been proposed as the basis for congenital diverticula.[13]

Routh postulated an infectious etiology in 1890.[14] He suggested that infection could result in obstruction of the paraurethral glands and in abscess formation. The resulting retention cyst might then rupture into the urethral lumen, creating a urethral diverticulum. Huffman's classic description of urethral anatomy in 1948[15] helped to support this theory. Meticulous dissection of 11 female cadavers, including the creation of paraffin molds of the urethra, revealed a considerably more complex anatomy of the paraurethral glands than previously suspected. Not only were there arbor-like branches to the paraurethral glands, but cystic dilation and inflammatory reaction were common, which helped to support the infectious basis for urethral diverticula formation. Gonococcus, *Escherichia coli*, and *Chlamydia* appear to be the common offending organisms.[16] Stasis and chronic infection also predispose to stone formation; they occur in 1.5–10% of urethral diverticula and may also increase the risk of carcinogenesis, although carcinoma within diverticula is rare.[10]

Urethral trauma has also been proposed as a potential etiology of urethral diverticula. Trauma could be due to repeated catheterizations, urethral dilations, or surgery to the anterior vaginal wall.[16] Similarly, parturition has been proposed as an etiology, although clearly it is not a universal etiology as an estimated 20% of women with urethral diverticula are nulliparous.[6]

PRESENTATION

The symptomatology reported by women with urethral diverticula is diverse, as are the frequency of symptoms in the literature. Table 7.2 presents data from several large series.[17–22] Between 7% and 20% of women with diverticula are asymptomatic but the majority of patients present with multiple symptoms.[10] Symptoms can be broadly grouped into urinary incontinence and irritative voiding.

Table 7.2 Presenting symptoms with urethral diverticula

Symptom	Range of reported frequency (%)
Incontinence	
Stress incontinence	9–70
Urge incontinence	4–35
Postvoid dribble	13–90
Irritative voiding	
Dysuria	10–80
Frequency	42–100
Urethral pain	26–45
Hematuria	7–35
Recurrent urinary tract infection	23–80

Leach and Bavendam[10] report that almost one third of their series of 37 women presented for urinary incontinence alone and in these women the diverticulum was identified during the evaluation for incontinence. The size of the diverticular ostia may determine the associated symptomatology. Large-necked diverticula are more apt to produce symptoms related to urinary incontinence, while small-necked diverticula will produce more irritative voiding symptoms. This latter category should include recurrent urinary tract infection, as this is a common presentation. The distinction between incontinence symptoms and irritative voiding symptoms may be helpful in directing the diagnostic evaluation.

The classic physical findings for urethral diverticula are a suburethral mass noted on pelvic examination and the expression of discharge from the urethral meatus during urethral massage. Tabulation of the frequency of these physical findings from the literature demonstrates a wide variability, with a range of 12–89% for the suburethral mass and of 2–31% for urethral discharge.[3,10,21,22] Pyuria is common in women with urethral diverticula. In one series 100% of women with diverticula had pyuria, although only 40% had a positive urine culture.[20]

EVALUATION

Perhaps the most important aspect of successfully diagnosing a urethral diverticulum is the physician's suspicion that one may be present. This diagnosis should be entertained in the differential diagnosis of both urinary incontinence and irritative voiding symptoms. The physical examination in these circumstances should include an evaluation of the anterior vaginal wall to assess for the presence of a suburethral mass, as well as urethral massage to determine the presence of discharge from the urethral meatus. Even such a thorough history and examination may be inconclusive. Furthermore, additional information is desirable in planning the surgical management of a suspected urethral diverticulum.

The location of the urethral diverticulum within the urethral lumen is essential as it impacts the choice of surgical repair. Distal diverticula can usually be managed with a marsupialization procedure, a significantly less morbid technique than any of the transvaginal diverticulectomy techniques used for more proximal lesions. Earlier reports[23] suggested that the majority of diverticula occurred in the distal urethra, but more recent series reveal that more than half open into the middle third of the urethral lumen.[6,7,10,24] Diverticular architecture also has surgical implications. In addition to the size of the diverticular ostia, it is useful to know whether there is a single diverticulum with multiple openings, or multiple diverticula, which occur in up to one half of patients.[16] As previously stated, many women with diverticula complain of urinary incontinence. Leach and Bavendam[10] reported genuine stress incontinence in 33% of women with diverticula, and mixed urinary incontinence in 16%. Genuine stress incontinence may be due to urethral hypermobility or intrinsic sphincteric deficiency. The latter may be more common in women with diverticula if the disruption of the urethral mucous membrane and muscularis interferes with normal urethral coaptation.

There are several diagnostic modalities that have been advocated towards this end including radiologic tests, urodynamic investigations, and endoscopic techniques (Table 7.3). The utility of a given test will depend on the circumstances of the patient, but in general the test should confirm the presence of the diverticulum, establish its location in the urethral lumen, provide information regarding architectural complexity, and determine whether it coexists with other urethral pathology.

Table 7.3 Diagnostic modalities for evaluating suspected urethral diverticula

Technique	Diagnostic accuracy (%)
Radiologic techniques	
Voiding cystourethrography	65–77
Positive-pressure urethrography	90
Ultrasonography	
Transvaginal	90
Intraluminal	100
Urodynamics	
Urethral pressure profilometry	72
Endoscopy	
Urethroscopy	90

Radiologic techniques

Radiologic testing has played an important role in the history of urethral diverticula. The development of the double-balloon urethral catheter, by Davis and Cain and then by Tratner (C.R. Bard, Covenington, GA), made possible the positive-pressure urethrogram. Davis and Cain's initial report[4] illustrated the relative frequency of this malady and provided physicians with a technique to confirm the diagnosis. The triple-lumen, double-balloon urethral catheter isolates the urethral lumen between an intravesical balloon and a sliding balloon that is tamponaded against the external urethral meatus. Radiopaque dye is introduced through the third lumen, which empties into the urethra between the two balloons. The balloons effectively seal the urethral lumen, permitting the dye to be injected with sufficient pressure to fill the urethral diverticula. Positive-pressure urethrography has a reported accuracy in diagnosing urethral diverticula of 90%.[7] Disadvantages include the need for fluoroscopy and increased patient discomfort compared with other techniques.

Voiding cystourethrography is another commonly used radiologic technique for diagnosing urethral diverticula. The voiding cystourethrogram depends on chance filling of the diverticulum during voiding, which decreases the diagnostic accuracy to 65–77%.[7,25] Some physicians prefer the simpler, and better tolerated, voiding cystourethrogram to the positive-pressure urethrogram, arguing that any diverticulum that is large enough to be symptomatic should fill during normal voiding. This is supported by Leach and Bavendam's series of 37 women in whom positive-pressure urethrography enhanced the diagnostic value of voiding cystourethrography in only one patient.[10] While this may be true for diverticula that produce symptoms of incontinence or postmicturition dribbling, it may not be true for diverticula that produce irritative voiding symptoms. Consequently, this may not be the optimal evaluation for this latter group of patients.

Ultrasonography

Ultrasonography may be used to diagnose urethral diverticula as well. Proponents of the technique suggest that it is superior for demonstrating multiloculation and multiple diverticula.[26] In addition to transvaginal ultrasonography, endoluminal ultrasonography has been advocated at the time of surgery, and early reports suggest that it is more accurate than either transvaginal ultrasonography or positive-pressure urethrography.[27]

Urodynamics

The presence of a biphasic urethral pressure profile is yet another indicator of urethral diverticula. It has a reported diagnostic accuracy of 72–100%.[10,24] Summitt and Stovall[24] were careful to point out that while the diagnostic sensitivity was 100% in their series, the specificity was only 80%. This is unacceptable since this modality used alone would recommend surgical intervention for women who do not have urethral diverticula. Advocates of urethral pressure profilometry argue that the true value of the urethral pressure profile is in planning the surgical intervention, as the biphasic profile provides information about the location of the diverticular ostia with respect to the functional urethral sphincter muscle. Summitt and Stovall tested this hypothesis and reported[24] that the urethral pressure profile provided no new information over that provided by cystourethroscopy or voiding cystourethrography in planning surgical repair in a series of nine women with urethral diverticula. Additionally, they found that the pressure depression on the profile poorly represented the location of the diverticular ostia. The primary value of urodynamics in women with urethral diverticula appears to be in diagnosing concurrent genuine stress incontinence.

Urethroscopy

Urethroscopy provides many of the advantages of other diagnostic modalities in evaluating urethral diverticula, with several advantages. Urethroscopy is a simple brief evaluation that does not expose the patient or physician to radiation. Dynamic urethroscopy provides visualization of the diverticular ostia as well as its location with respect to the anatomic urethra. Because the irrigation can be instilled under pressure, even the smallest diverticulum can be identified. The reported accuracy is 80–100%.[7,10,24] It is readily available to physicians evaluating urinary incontinence, as approximately one third of women with urethral diverticula present with primary complaints of urinary incontinence. Moreover, it provides additional information about urethral hypermobility and urethrovesical junction coaptation.

ENDOSCOPIC TECHNIQUE

Robertson's original description of urethroscopy utilized carbon dioxide as a distending media. Sterile water and saline are easier distending media for most indications, but carbon dioxide may have some benefit in filling diverticula and demonstrating diverticular ostia.

The urethral meatus is cleansed with a disinfectant. With the carbon dioxide flowing, the urethroscope is introduced into the urethral meatus. The center of the urethral lumen is maintained in the center of the operator's visual field and the urethral lumen, distended by the carbon dioxide, is followed to the urethrovesical junction. The urethral mucosa is examined for redness, pallor, exudate, and polyps as the urethroscope is advanced.

Once the urethroscope is in the bladder, the urethrovesical junction is obstructed with a vaginal finger to allow the bladder to fill. After a bladder volume of approximately 250 ml is achieved, the urethroscope is withdrawn into the proximal urethral lumen and the urethroscope is gradually withdrawn. The vaginal finger obstructs the urethral lumen proximal to the urethroscope to maximize distension of the urethral lumen, and massages the urethra to demonstrate exudate (see Fig. 3.2). The urethroscope should be maintained in the center of the urethral lumen to provide the best possible view of the urethral mucosa. The ostia of diverticula, like the urethral glands (Plate 1.9), are the most commonly seen on the posterior surface of the urethral lumen, but may be found on the anterior wall as well. Gentle massage of the urethra against the scope milks exudate from diverticular openings, which helps to localize the ostia (Plate 3.7). When diverticula are identified, the location with respect to the urethrovesical junction and external meatus should be noted as they can occur in the proximal (Plate 3.6), mid (Plate 3.7), or distal urethra. The endoscopist should look for multiple diverticula (Plate 3.8) and diverticula with multiple or complex openings (Plate 3.5).

REFERENCES

1. Hey W. *Practical Observations in Surgery*. Philadelphia: J Humphries, 1805.
2. Novack R. Editorial comment. *Obstet Gynecol Surv* 1953; **8**: 423.
3. Davis HJ, Telinde RW. Urethral diverticula: an assay of 100 cases. *J Urol* 1958; **80**: 34–9.
4. Davis HJ, Cain LG. Positive pressure urethrography: a new diagnostic method. *J Urol* 1956; **75**: 753–8.
5. Anderson MJF. The incidence of diverticula in the female urethra. *J Urol* 1967; **98**: 96–9.
6. Lee RA. Diverticulum of the urethra: clinical representation, diagnosis, and management. *Clin Obstet Gynecol* 1984; **27**: 490–5.
7. Robertson JR. Urethral diverticula. In: Ostergard DR, Bent AE (eds) *Urogynecology and Urodynamics: Theory and Practice*. Baltimore: Williams and Wilkins, 1996: 361–70.
8. Benjamin J, Elliot L, Cooper JF, Bjornson L. Urethral diverticulum in adult females. *Urology* 1974; **3**: 1–7.
9. Davis BL, Robinson DG. Diverticula of the female urethra: assay of 120 cases. *J Urol* 1970; **104**: 850–4.
10. Leach GE, Bavendam TG. Female urethral diverticula. *Urology* 1987; **30**: 407–15.
11. Glassman TA, Weinerth JL, Glenn JF. Neonatal female urethral diverticulum. *Urology* 1975; **5**: 249–53.
12. Marshall S. Urethral diverticula in young girls. *Urology* 1981; **17**: 243–7.

13. Ginsburg DS, Genadry R. Suburethral diverticulum in the female. *Obstet Gynecol Surv* 1984; **39**: 1–9.
14. Routh A. Urethral diverticula. *BMJ* 1890; **i**: 361.
15. Huffman JW. Detailed anatomy of the paraurethral ducts in adult human female. *Am J Obstet Gynecol* 1948; **55**: 86–92.
16. Drutz HP. Urethral diverticula. *Obstet Gynecol Clin North Am* 1989; **16**: 923–9.
17. Hoffman M, Adams W. Recognition and repair of urethral diverticula. *Am J Obstet Gynecol* 1965; **92**: 106–11.
18. Kittredge R, Bienstock M, Finby N. Urethral diverticula in women. *AJR Am J Roentgenol Radium Ther Nucl Med* 1966; **98**: 200–4.
19. MacKinnon M, Pratt JH, Pool TL. Diverticulum of the female urethra. *Surg Clin North Am* 1959; **39**: 953–62.
20. Rozesahegyi J, Magasi P, Szule E. Diverticulum of the female urethra: a report of 50 cases. *Acta Chir Hung* 1984; **15**: 33–9.
21. Pathak UN, House MJ. Diverticulum of the female urethra. *Obstet Gynecol* 1970; **36**: 789–93.
22. Woodhouse CRJ, Flynn JT, Molland EA, Blandy JP. Urethral diverticulum in females. *Br J Urol* 1980; **52**: 305–9.
23. Menville JG, Mitchell JD. Diverticulum of the female urethra. *J Urol* 1944; **51**: 411–14.
24. Summitt RL, Stovall TG. Urethral diverticula: evaluation by urethral pressure profilometry, cystourethroscopy, and voiding cystourethrogram. *Obstet Gynecol* 1992; **80**: 695–9.
25. Houser LM, VonEschenbach AC. Diverticula of the female urethra: diagnostic importance of post-voiding film. *Urology* 1987; **3**: 453–5.
26. Lee TG, Keller FS. Urethral diverticulum: diagnosis by ultrasound. *AJR Am J Roentgenol* 1977; **128**: 690–4.
27. Chancellor MB, Liu JB, Rivas DA, Karasick S, Bagley DH, Goldberg BB. Intraoperative endoluminal ultrasound evaluation of urethral diverticula. *J Urol* 1995; **153**: 72–5.

URETHRAL DIVERTICULA

CHAPTER 8

Urinary tract fistula

Alfred E. Bent

Risk factors

Presentations

Diagnosis

RISK FACTORS

In developed countries most urogenital fistulas (Table 8.1) are secondary to gynecologic surgery, and most of these are vesico-vaginal fistulas secondary to hysterectomy for menorrhagia, uterine fibroids, and pelvic relaxation.[1] These typically occur by post-operative day 1–10 in two thirds of patients, by day 11–20 in one third, and by day 21–30 in less than 5% of cases. Other etiologies include congenital causes (rare), trauma from childbirth in developing countries, inflammatory (long-term indwelling urethral catheter, foreign body, tuberculosis, schistosomiasis) and neoplastic (cancer of the cervix and bladder).[2] Risk factors (Table 8.2) in these cases include preoperative radiation, pelvic inflammatory disease, previous surgery, and endometriosis.[3] Radiation-induced fistulas most frequently follow treatment for cancer of the cervix, and these can take years to develop.

Ureterovaginal fistulas are most frequently secondary to hysterectomy, especially radical hysterectomy. Urethrovaginal fistulas are predominant in developing countries as a result of obstetric causes. In developed countries this fistula generally follows elective urethral and vaginal operations, urethral trauma, and radiation treatment[4,5] (Table 8.3).

The four most common vesicoenteric fistulas are colovesical, rectovesical, ileovesical, and appendicovesical. The common causes of this rare condition include diverticulitis (50–70%), malignancy (20%), Crohn's disease (10%), and trauma (iatrogenic, foreign body, pelvic fracture). Vesicouterine fistulas are usually secondary to cesarean section where suture repair for the uterus is placed through the bladder, or following uterine rupture related to precipitate

---

Table 8.1 Fistulas of the lower urinary tract

Vesicovaginal
Urethrovaginal
Enterovesical
Vesicouterine
Vesicocervical

Table 8.2 Risk factors for fistula

Previous radiation
Pelvic inflammatory disease
Previous surgery
Endometriosis
Cancer

Table 8.3 Causes of urethrovaginal fistula

Obstetric injury
  Prolonged labor
  Forceps application and delivery
  Precipitate delivery

Secondary to inflammation or surgery for urethral diverticulum
  Spontaneous rupture into vagina
  Incision of abscessed diverticulum
  Nonhealing after surgery (hematoma, poor blood supply)

Complication of anterior colporrhaphy
  Local infection
  Impaired blood supply
  Constricting sutures
  Hematoma
  Suture in urethral lumen
  Urethral injury not recognized
  Repeated catheterizations after operation

Resection of bladder neck

Other
  Malignant change
  Radiation
  Venereal disease
  Trauma

delivery. Other causes include curettage, intrauterine catheter placement, or high forceps delivery.

PRESENTATIONS

The clinical presentation of vesicovaginal fistula is continuous leakage of urine from the vagina. An early clinical sign is unsuspected postoperative hematuria after 48 hours. Most ureterovaginal fistulas are leaking urine in 14 days or less from the time of injury. Other clinical features include unexplained abdominal pain, abdominal mass, or fever. The clinical presentation of urethrovaginal fistula is with urine leakage from the vagina upon standing (usually immediately after injury), upon catheter removal or within 2 weeks of surgery on or near the urethra, or somewhat delayed in cases of radiation injury.[1]

In the case of vesicoenteric fistula, many present with suprapubic pain and chronic urinary tract infection. Passage of urine may be seen through the rectum. Pneumaturia occurs in 60% of patients, and fecaluria is very uncommon but is pathognomonic of fistula.[2] The clinical presentation of vesicouterine fistula is with cyclic hematuria,[6] while vesicocervical fistula may present with menstrual hematuria

Table 8.4. Diagnostic modalities

Confirm presence of fistula
    Pyridium staining of urine
    Exclude loss from urethra

Localization of source – bladder, urethra, or other
    Tampon test
    Flat tire test
    Urethrocystoscopy

Imaging techniques
    Intravenous pyelography
    Cystography (voiding)
    Barium enema

where a flap-type tract permits fluid to pass only from the uterus to the bladder.

DIAGNOSIS

Diagnosis is made in three steps after suspicion leads to consideration of the presence of a fistula (Table 8.4). Step one is to confirm that watery drainage is urine, and pyridium may be used for this purpose. The next step is to exclude urinary incontinence occurring from the urethra by filling the bladder and observing loss from the urethra or vagina. Finally the source of the fistula needs to be found.[7] This commences with a thorough speculum inspection which may reveal a fistulous site to the vagina. The flat tire test may also be performed. Water is placed in the vagina and carbon dioxide gas is infused into the bladder. As the vaginal fornices are observed, the fistula site can be seen bubbling from the bladder (Figure 8.1).

The double-contrast test is performed by filling the bladder with 1% carmine and injecting 5 ml indigo carmine intravenously. The vagina is packed with gauze sponges. Red staining on the outlet sponge suggests leakage from the urethra, red staining on the middle vaginal sponge suggests vesicovaginal fistula, and a blue stain on the upper sponge implies ureterovaginal fistula. Cystoscopy is the most useful test and may allow visualization of the fistula site in the bladder (Plate 6.1). A posthysterectomy vesicovaginal fistula on the bladder side appears above the trigone medial to the ureters (Plate 6.2). At vaginoscopy it is at the vaginal vault (Plate 6.3). Cystoscopy may show edema and congestion, or even mucosal papillomatous hyperplasia in enterovesical fistula. A barium enema may exclude bowel conditions. Other adjuncts include urethroscopy for urethrovaginal fistulas (Plates 6.4 and 6.5), retrograde pyelography, intravenous pyelography, cystography, and voiding cystourethrography.

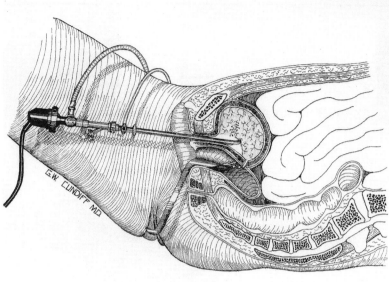

Fig. 8.1 Flat tire test. Water or saline is placed into the vaginal fornix. The cystoscope is advanced into the bladder using carbon dioxide as a distending medium. The vaginal fistula site is identified as the bubbles of carbon dioxide gas are seen passing from the bladder into the vagina. The vesical fistula site is observed with the cystoscope

Sometimes a ureteral catheter can be passed into a visible fistula opening, and contrast injected to outline its path.

REFERENCES

1. Lee RA. Management of genitourinary fistulas. In Hurt WG (ed.) *Urogynecologic Surgery.* Gaithersburg: Aspen, 1993: 131–8.
2. Lang EK, Fritzsche. Fistulas of the genitourinary tract. In Pollack HM (ed.) *Clinical Urography.* Philadelphia: WB Saunders, 1990: 2579–93.
3. Singh A, Marshall FF. Urinary fistulas. In Gillenwater JY, Grayhack JT, Howards SS, Duckett JW (eds) *Adult and Pediatric Urology,* 2nd edn. St Louis: Mosby–Year Book, 1987: 1119–34.
4. Elkins TE, Fitzpatrick C. Lower urinary tract fistulas. In Walters MD, Karram MM (eds). St Louis: Mosby–Year Book, 1993: 330–41.
5. Gray LA. Urethrovaginal fistulas and fistulas of the urethrovesical junction. In Slate WG (ed.) *Disorders of the Female Urethra and Urinary Incontinence,* 2nd edn. Baltimore: Williams and Wilkins, 1982: 234–41.
6. Nichols DH, Randall CL. Vesicovaginal and other urogenital fistulas. In Nichols DH, Randall CL (eds) *Vaginal Surgery,* 4th edn. Baltimore: Williams and Wilkins, 1996: 433–60.
7. Raz S, Little NA, Juma S. Female urology. In Walsh PC, Retik AB, Stamey TA, Vaughan ED Jr (eds) *Campbell's Urology,* 6th edn. Philadelphia: WB Saunders, 1992: 2782–828.

CHAPTER 9

Perioperative evaluation of vesical and ureteral integrity

Geoffrey W. Cundiff

Table 9.1 Incidence of ureteral injury during major gynecologic surgery

Reference	Year	*n*	Prevalence
Samson[1]	1902	955	1.5
Herman et al.[4]	1946	7966	0.05
St Martin et al.[5]	1953	332	2.4
Conger et al.[6]	1954	2290	0.6
Mann et al.[7]	1988	3185	0.4
Stanhope et al.[8]	1991	5379	0.3
Wiskind and Thompson[3]	1995	1270	0.005

INCIDENCE OF URINARY TRACT INJURY

The incidence of operative injury to the lower urinary tract has not changed significantly since Samson[1] reviewed the subject in 1902. The majority of ureteral injuries today occur during gynecologic operations, and lower urinary tract injury is one of the most frequent reasons for medical litigation against gynecologists.[2,3] Estimates for the incidence of injury to the ureters during major gynecologic surgery ranges from 0.4 to 2.5% (Table 9.1).[1,3–8]

The incidence of lower urinary tract injury is still higher for urogynecologic surgery. Harris et al.[9] recently reported an incidence of lower urinary tract injury of 5.7% during reconstructive surgery for incontinence or prolapse. Importantly, 4% were injuries unrecognized before urinary tract endoscopy. These included three bladder injuries and six ureteral injuries. The procedures most commonly associated with urinary tract injury were retropubic urethropexy and uterosacral ligament plication for vault suspension (McCall's stitch). The uterosacral plication and sutures for elevation of the bladder neck were also identified by Stanhope et al.[8] as well as by Pettit and Petrou[10] as procedures frequently associated with ureteral obstruction.

PREVENTION

Approaches to prevent ureteral compromise during pelvic surgery are listed in Table 9.2. A complete understanding of pelvic anatomy and good surgical technique are the best approaches to prevent damage to the lower urinary tract during pelvic surgery. Spence and Boone[11] recommended identification of the course of the ureter to

Table 9.2 Techniques to prevent ureteral injury during pelvic surgery

Preoperative excretory urography
Preoperative ureteral catheterization
Intraoperative ureteral identification

prevent its injury during pelvic surgery in 1961, and this approach has been shown to decrease ureteral injury from an abdominal approach.[8,10–12] Palpation of the ureter is also possible from the vaginal approach in 90% of patients, but is used infrequently.[12]

As important as a complete knowledge of pelvic anatomy in general, and of the course of the ureters specifically, is to protecting the lower urinary tract, intraoperative ureteral identification or palpation is not reliable in the presence of fibrotic or fixed pelvic disease. This is particularly true of the most vulnerable distal ureter. Moreover, palpation does not prevent injuries to the bladder.

The shortcomings of intraoperative ureteral palpation have led some to advocate preoperative measures to clarify the course of the ureters. Excretory urography is one such technique.[13,15] While preoperative urography can identify congenital anomalies and intrinsic urinary tract disease, studies show that the two-dimensional image does not facilitate ureteral identification at the operating table.[13]

Preoperative ureteral catheterization has also been advocated to prevent intraoperative ureteral injury. Unfortunately, the technique is probably not useful to prevent ureteral injury during the majority of pelvic operations.[14] This fact was recognized by Symmonds[15] who identified several shortcomings of routine preoperative ureteral catheterization. Firstly, the use of ureteral catheters during all pelvic operations is unnecessarily invasive, yet accurate identification of patients most at risk of ureteral damage is impossible because most injuries occur during straightforward hysterectomy. Moreover, ureteral catheters do not facilitate the identification of the distal ureter in the presence of pelvic fibrotic pathology. Universal ureteral catheterization also subjects patients to mucosal trauma and spasm of the ureter. Perhaps most importantly, catheterizing of the ureter with a firm non-yielding catheter may actually predispose to trauma during dissection by fixing the ureter against a hard surface. While ureteral catheterization is a valuable tool for evaluating and managing damage to the ureters, it is not generally warranted prophylactically. Ureteral markers can be useful, however, during any operation with a high potential for ureteral injury, including patients requiring radical surgery and those with abnormal pelvic anatomy.

INTRAOPERATIVE EVALUATION

The venial sin is injury to the ureter, but the mortal sin is failure of recognition.[14]

Higgin's declaration in 1967 still pertains. Since prevention of lower urinary tract injury is not achieved by preoperative radiologic

Table 9.3 Techniques to evaluate lower urinary tract integrity during surgery

Bladder integrity
Intentional cystotomy
Endoscopic techniques
    Cystoscopy
    Suprapubic teloscopy

Ureteral integrity
Indigo carmine
Ureteral catheterization

imaging, or preoperative placement of ureteral catheters, and even careful intraoperative identification of the course of the ureters does not insure lower urinary tract integrity, measures must be taken following surgery to prevent the patient from leaving the operating theatre with an unrecognized injury. Since 15–31% of ureteral injuries are asymptomatic, the time for evaluation of lower urinary tract integrity is during surgery.[5,6] Different approaches to evaluating lower urinary tract integrity at the time of surgery are listed in Table 9.3. Bladder integrity can be assessed either by intentional cystotomy or by endoscopic techniques. Many surgeons are reluctant to incise the bladder without clear indication owing to the need for closure and the associated delay in voiding. Endoscopy, from either a transurethral or suprapubic approach, is therefore the preferred technique of evaluating the lower urinary tract for many pelvic surgeons.[3,11] Regardless of whether a cystotomy or endoscopy is used to evaluate the bladder integrity, ureteral function should be evaluated as well either by noting the efflux of urine or, in its absence, by ureteral catheterization.

POSTOPERATIVE CYSTOSCOPY

Indications

A variety of algorithms have been advocated for determining patients who should undergo evaluation of the lower urinary tract after pelvic surgery. The higher incidence of injury during vaginal culdoplasty and urethropexy has already been stated, but injuries also occur with other reconstructive operations including anterior colporrhaphy, paravaginal defect repair, and abdominal culdoplasty. Moreover, demographic and intraoperative parameters are not predictive of who will suffer injury.[9] Consequently, several authors have advocated endoscopic evaluation of the lower urinary tract after all reconstructive surgery.[3,9] Other surgeons reserve endoscopic evaluation of the lower urinary tract for patients with difficult dissections or neoplastic or fibrotic disease that precludes adequate ureteral identification and palpation. While pursuing injury based on the surgeon's suspicion or for procedures with an increased risk of jeopardizing the lower urinary tract seems sound, it may miss a significant number of injuries. As Symmonds[15] noted, the majority of genitourinary fistulas occur after straightforward total hysterectomy for benign indications.

Technique

The approach to assessment of the integrity of the bladder mucosa following pelvic surgery is similar to that described for diagnostic cystoscopy (see Chapter 3). A thorough survey of the bladder is made with special attention to the portions of the bladder that are potentially jeopardized by the given procedure (see Fig. 3.3). Inspection of the anteriolateral aspects of the mucosa is important after a retropubic urethropexy, whereas inspection of the trigone is warranted following a difficult vaginal hysterectomy or dissection of an anterior enterocele sac from the bladder. An assessment of ureteral integrity is warranted after any retropubic suspension or culdoplasty, but is also warranted in any case where there is a suspicion of ureteral injury. Visualization of the ureteral orifice during efflux is sufficient, and is facilitated by intravenous administration of indigo carmine (5 ml) approximately 5 minutes before initiating cystoscopy (Plate 7.1). Efflux of indigo carmine is usually visible in 5–10 minutes but sometimes takes up to 20 minutes. For patients with curtailed renal function, a loop diuretic, such as furosemide, can be helpful to hasten ureteral efflux. The absence of efflux is an indication for the passage of ureteral catheters to evaluate for potential obstruction.

URETERAL CATHETERIZATION

Indications

In the absence of ureteral efflux of indigo carmine-stained urine, ureteral catheterization is useful to confirm the possible obstruction. It adds minimal time to the procedure as the cystoscope is already in place. Additionally, it provides valuable information regarding the level of obstruction with respect to the ureteral orifice and bladder. Ureteral catheterization can also be used to place ureteral markers before surgery in which difficult pelvic pathology is anticipated.

Ureteral catheters

The most useful catheter for evaluating potential ureteral obstruction is the general purpose or whistle-tip catheter. Refer to Chapter 10 for a more indepth discussion of ureteral catheters.

Technique

Either a 30° or 70° angled scope should be used for ureteral catheterization. An Albarran bridge facilitates ureteral catheterization but is not essential to its completion. The telescope is oriented to view the bladder base, and the ureteral catheter is advanced into the field of view. The ureteral orifice is located and the catheter tip is oriented in the axis of the ureteral lumen. The tip is threaded into the ureteral orifice by advancing the entire cystoscope. Once the tip passes the ureteral orifice, the catheter is gently advanced until it meets resistance as it passes into the renal pelvis, which is generally 25–30 cm.

Difficulty in passing the catheter may be due to a surgical obstruction but anatomic variation, mucosal fold, or ureteral tortuousity should be considered as well. A stenotic orifice is suspected in the presence of immediate resistance to the catheter tip. A smaller caliber catheter and slight withdrawal of the catheter tip into the sheath to minimize its bending will often overcome the stenosis. A mucosal fold can be negotiated by repositioning the patient, bladder, or cystoscope. Trendelenburg positioning helps to alter the position of the intramural ureter, as does further filling or emptying of the bladder. A filiform-tip catheter is also valuable for negotiating strictures or ureteral tortuousity.

Gentle technique is essential to preventing hematuria and resulting ureteral colic. Other potential complications include perforation and ureteral spasm, but with proper technique the risk of complications is minimal.

SUPRAPUBIC TELESCOPY

Indications

Transurethral cystoscopy is well suited to evaluating vesical and ureteral integrity when pelvic surgery is performed from a vaginal approach but is inconvenient in conjunction with an abdominal approach. Valuable operating time is lost by closing the abdominal wound to permit repositioning and prepping for transurethral cystoscopy. Moreover, any significant cystoscopic findings mandate reopening the abdomen for surgical correction. In spite of these inconveniences, the majority of ureteral injuries occur during abdominal pelvic surgery.[16] Suprapubic telescopy addresses this dilemma by providing a method to perform endoscopy from an abdominal approach.[17] Due to the simplicity of the technique, suprapubic telescopy compares favorably to the alternatives of open cystotomy or dissection of ureters in terms of required operating time and morbidity. Moreover, it is an easy transition for an endoscopist experienced at transurethral cystoscopy.

Technique

Suprapubic telescopy (Fig. 9.1) is an extraperitoneal technique that begins with closure of the anterior peritoneum to prevent contamination of the peritoneal cavity with spilled urine and subsequent vesicoperitoneal fistulas. If indigo carmine is to be used to help identify the ureteral orifices, it should be given at this juncture to permit time for renal excretion. The bladder cavity is filled through a transurethral Foley catheter to at least 400 ml. This is simplified by placing a triple-lumen Foley catheter before the beginning of the operation.

A 1–2-cm purse-string suture is placed into the muscularis layer of

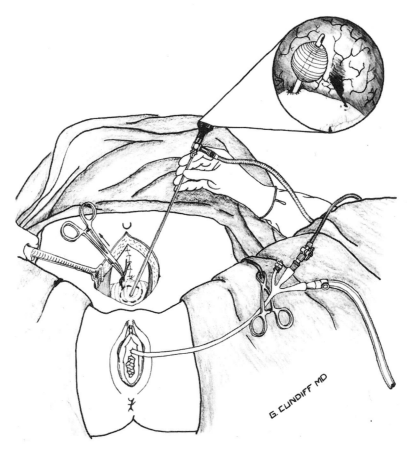

Fig. 9.1 Suprapubic telescopy. The bladder is filled retrogradely through a transurethral triple-lumen Foley catheter to a volume of 400 ml. A 1–2-cm purse-string absorbable suture is placed into the muscularis layer of the dome of the bladder and a stab incision is made within the purse-string for insertion of the telescope. The purse-string is tightened sufficiently to prevent leakage without limiting movement of the telescope. Orientation can be achieved by identifying the transurethral Foley catheter bulb. The trigone is beneath the bulb with the urethral and ureteral orifices at its apices

the dome of the bladder, using a 2–0 absorbable suture. To facilitate introduction of the telescope, two stay sutures can be placed within the purse-string using similar suture material but with a full-thickness purchase. A stab incision made between the stay sutures provides an opening for insertion of the telescope. Since distension of the bladder is achieved through the transurethral catheter, the sheath and bridge are not necessary, and only the telescope is inserted. The purse-string is tightened sufficiently to prevent leakage without limiting the movement of the telescope.

A 30° telescope provides the best view of the trigone and ureteral orifices while also permitting a thorough bladder survey. Orientation can be achieved by identifying the transurethral Foley catheter bulb. The trigone is beneath the bulb with the urethral and ureteral orifices at its apices. In the event that ureteral catheterization is planned, a sheath with a sufficient irrigation–working channel can be used with the telescope. If suprapubic catheterization is planned, the catheter can be placed through the same stab incision when telescopy is completed.

REFERENCES

1. Samson JA. Ligation and clamping of the ureter as complications of surgical operations. *Am Med* 1902; **4**: 693.
2. Dowling RA, Corrieve JN, Sandler CM. Iatrogenic ureteral injury. *J Urol* 1986; **135**: 912.
3. Wiskind AK, Thompson JD. Should cystoscopy be performed at every gynecologic operation to diagnose unsuspected ureteral injury? *J Pelvic Surg* 1995; **1**: 134–7.
4. Herman L, Green LB, Hayllar BL. Ureteral injuries. *J Urol* 1946; **56**: 688–96.
5. St Martin EC. Ureteral injury in gynecologic surgery. *J Urol* 1953; **70**: 51–7.
6. Conger K, Beecham CT, Horrax TM. Ureteral injury in pelvic surgery: current thought on incidence, pathogenesis, prophylaxis and treatment. *Obstet Gynecol* 1954; **3**: 343–57.
7. Mann WJ, Arato M, Patsner B, Stone ML. Ureteral injuries in an obstetrics and gynecology training program: etiology and management. *Obstet Gynecol* 1988; **72**: 82–5.
8. Stanhope CR, Wilson TO, Utz WJ, Smith LH, O'Brien PC. Suture entrapment and secondary ureteral obstruction. *Am J Obstet Gynecol* 1991; **164**: 1513–19.
9. Harris RL, Cundiff GW, Theofrastous JP, Yoon H, Bump RC, Addison WA. The value of intraoperative cystoscopy in urogynecologic and reconstructive surgery. *Am J Obstet Gynecol* 1997; **177**: 1367–71.
10. Pettit PD, Petrou SP. The value of cystoscopy in major vaginal surgery. *Obstet Gynecol* 1994; **84**: 318–20.
11. Spence HM, Boone T. Surgical injuries to the ureter. *JAMA* 1961; **176**: 1070–6.
12. Lee RA, Symmonds RE, Williams TJ. Current status of genitourinary fistula. *Obstet Gynecol* 1988; **72**: 313–19.
13. Piscitelli JT, Simel DL, Addison WA. Who should have intravenous pyelograms before hysterectomy for benign disease? *Obstet Gynecol* 1987; **69**: 541–5.
14. Higgins CC. Ureteral injuries during surgery. *JAMA* 1967; **199**: 118–24.
15. Symmonds RE. Ureteral injuries associated with gynecologic surgery: prevention and management. *Clin Obstet Gynecol* 1976; **19**: 623–44.
16. Freda VC, Tacchi D. Ureteral injury discovered after pelvic surgery. *Am J Obstet Gynecol* 1962; **85**: 406–9.
17. Timmons MC, Addison WA. Suprapubic telescopy: extraperitoneal intraoperative technique to demonstrate ureteral patency. *Obstet Gynecol* 1990; **75**: 137–9.

CHAPTER 10

Operative urethrocystoscopy

Geoffrey W. Cundiff

INTRODUCTION

The most common applications of cystourethroscopy in gynecology use the endoscope in a diagnostic capacity. Operative uses of endoscopy in the female lower urinary tract include diagnostic techniques modified for use during gynecologic surgery, minor operative procedures performed through an operative cystoscope, and ureteral catheterization.

INTRAOPERATIVE PROCEDURES

Cystoscopy is an important element of surgery of the female genitourinary system. It is commonly used to judge coaptation during periurethral injections (see Chapter 11), to assess the elevation of the urethrovesical junction during urethropexy procedures, to facilitate surgical repair of urinary tract fistula (see Chapter 8) and urethral diverticula (see Chapter 7), to insure the safe placement of suprapubic catheters, and to evaluate the ureters and bladder mucosa for inadvertent damage (see Chapter 9).

Periurethral injections

Cystoscopy is essential to both the periurethral and transurethral techniques of placing periurethral bulking agents. Visualization of the urethral lumen with the urethroscope allows the surgeon to advance the needle to the proper position just lateral to the urethrovesical junction. It also permits injection of sufficient material to achieve coaptation without breaching the urethral mucosa. Techniques for placing periurethral bulking agents are described in detail in Chapter 11.

Endoscopic urethropexy

As part of his modification of the needle urethropexy, Stamey[1] advocated utilization of a cystoscope to insure correct suture placement and avoid bladder injuries. Cystoscopy is now commonly used during needle urethropexy to assess the elevation of the urethrovesical junction as well as to insure that the needle has not breached the integrity of bladder mucosa. Similarly, an endoscopic evaluation of the urethrovesical junction is used by some surgeons during retropubic urethropexy, and suburethral sling (Plates 7.2 and 7.3). A recent report suggests that the intraoperative endoscopic view of the bladder neck is neither reproducible nor predictive of postoperative success.[2] The same investigation also showed that other commonly used techniques to assess the elevation of the urethrovesical junction, including the urethral angle as assessed by a urethral cotton swab and measuring the distance from the urethrovesical junction to the symphysis pubis, were equally unpredictive of postoperative pressure transmission. This emphasizes the importance of surgical experience when judging the ideal elevation of the urethrovesical junction, regardless of which technique is used. In contrast to the other methods, cystoscopy also permits an intraoperative evaluation for damage to the ureters and bladder mucosa, which is discussed in Chapter 9.

Suprapubic catheter placement

Cystoscopy increases the safety of suprapubic catheter placement using the suprapubic stab technique. It facilitates intelligent insertion by confirming proper orientation and providing visualization of the entry. It also guarantees proper final positioning of the catheter.[3]

Before using the suprapubic stab technique of catheter placement, the patient should be in Trendelenburg position with greater than 400 ml of bladder volume. The trocar is directed towards the bladder dome two finger breadths above the symphysis pubis, and pierces the bladder mucosa under direct visualization. The catheter should also be anchored in place, either with a suture or balloon, while the tip is visualized in the bladder cavity.

OFFICE PROCEDURES

Urogynecologists generally leave the majority of operative cystoscopy to urologists. There are, however, several minor procedures that are easily performed in the office during diagnostic cystoscopy. These include biopsy of mucosal lesions and removal of small foreign bodies including bladder stones and intravesical sutures. These procedures can generally be performed in an outpatient setting but, because they require a larger cystoscope sheath (>22F) and may cause some patient discomfort, anesthesia is recommended.

Anesthesia

Intravesical instillation of anesthetic is often sufficient but can be augmented by a bladder pillar block. For bladder installation, the bladder is catheterized and drained. Some 50 ml 4% Lidocaine solution is instilled and left in place for 5 minutes. The bladder pillar block can be placed while waiting to drain the instilled Lidocaine from the bladder. The block is performed by injecting 5 ml 1%

Lidocaine solution 3 mm submucosally at the bladder pillars. After placement of a bi-valve speculum, the bladder pillars are located in the lateral fornices at 2 and 10 o'clock with respect to the cervix. If the uterus is absent, placement of a Sims speculum reveals the location of the bladder pillars on the anterior vaginal wall just superior and lateral to the urethrovesical junction.[4]

Operative technique

Operative cystoscopy requires a larger diameter sheath that will accommodate the instrument in the operative channel. A 22F sheath is generally sufficient. Operative sheaths often have two operative ports for passage of instruments and a 22F sheath will permit the passage of two instruments that are 4F or less. With the exception of ureteral catheters, two ports are rarely necessary.

Due to the focal length of the optics, the best view is immediately in front of the telescope and this is where operative procedures should take place. Following introduction of the cystoscope into the bladder and instillation of a sufficient volume to view the entire vesical wall, the instrument is introduced into the operative port and advanced until it is visible just at the end of the cystoscope. Gross movements should be made by moving the cystoscope while minor adjustments are made by moving the instrument itself (Fig. 10.1). This approach keeps the operation in the optimal field of view. Irrigation at a brisk rate helps to keep the field from being obscured by hemorrhage.

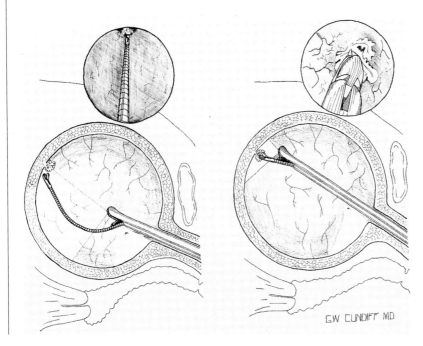

G.W. CUNDIFF MD

Fig. 10.1 Operating through a cystoscope. **a.** Incorrect technique: all movements are made with the instrument in the operative port, while the cystoscope is stabilized. **b.** Correct technique: the cystoscope is used to make gross adjustments while the instrument is moved for fine adjustments

The bleeding that occurs with biopsy will usually stop by itself, although the patient should be apprised of potential minor hematuria immediately after the procedure. If excessive hemorrhage occurs, this can be controlled by electrocautery utilizing a flexible monopolar electrode with a nonelectrolyte irrigant.

URETERAL CATHETERIZATION

Catheterizing the ureteral orifices has been a goal of the endoscopist since the early cystoscopes of the nineteenth century. With today's technology, catheterization is accomplished with ease and safety. In gynecology, the primary indications for ureteral catheterization are evaluating potential ureteral obstruction and the placement of ureteral markers. Ureteral markers are useful for any surgery with a high potential for ureteral injury, including radical surgery and surgery with abnormal pelvic anatomy. They are also used for retrograde pyelography.

Ureteral catheters are available in various sizes and with a number of specialized tips (Table 10.1). Although available from 3 to 12F, the most useful catheter calibers are in the 4–7F range. The most common catheters are the general-purpose catheter and the whistle-tip catheter. Specialized tips include the spiral filiform for negotiating strictures and curves, and the acorn tip for retrograde pyelography (Fig. 10.2). Catheters are fabricated from plastic or Dacron (Du Pont, Wilmington, Delaware, USA) and are generally radio-opaque. They also have graduated centimeter markings for judging the length of insertion.

Once the ureteral orifice is located, the ureteral catheter is advanced into the field of view. Although the deflecting mechanism of the Albarran bridge facilitates ureteral catheterization, it is usually not essential to its completion. The catheter is placed just outside the

Table 10.1 Ureteral catheters by function

Ureteral markers
   General purpose
   Whistle tip

Strictures
   Filiform

Indwelling
   Double J

Retrograde pyelography
   Acorn tip
   Rutner tip

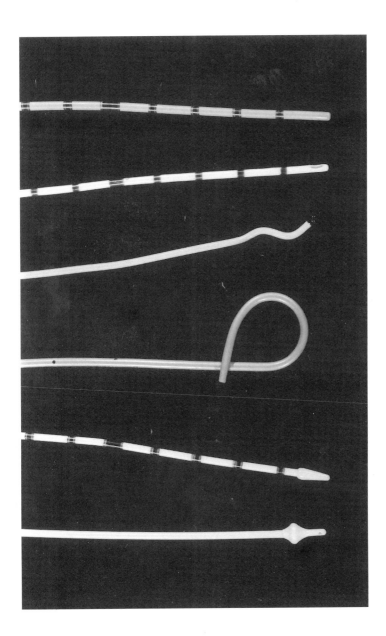

Fig. 10.2 Ureteral catheter tips. In descending order: general purpose, whistle tip, filiform, double J, acorn, Rutner

fenestrated end of the cystoscope with the catheter tip oriented in the axis of the ureteral lumen. The tip is threaded into the ureteral orifice by advancing the entire cystoscope. Once the tip passes the ureteral orifice, the catheter is gently advanced until it meets resistance as it passes into the renal pelvis, which is generally 25–30 cm.

If the catheter is to be left in place it should be secured to a transurethral catheter and connected to a drainage device. Gentle technique is essential to preventing hematuria and resulting colic. Other potential complications include perforation and ureteral spasm, but with proper methods the risk of complication is minimal.

REFERENCES

1. Stamey TA. Endoscopic suspension of the vesical neck for urinary incontinence. *Surg Gynecol Obstet* 1973; **136**: 547–54.
2. Bump RC, Hurt WG, Elser DM, Theofrastous JP, Fantl JA, McClish DK. Reliability of intra-operative anatomic, endoscopic, and urodynamic measurements and their correlation with post-operative pressure transmission in women undergoing bladder neck suspension surgery. *Neurourol Urodynam* 1995; **14**: 490–1.
3. Cundiff G, Bent AE. Suprapubic catheterization complicated by bowel injury. *Int J Urogynecol* 1995; **6**: 110–13.
4. Ostergard DR. Bladder pillar block anesthesia for urethral dilation in women. *Am J Obstet Gynecol* 1980; **136**: 187–8.

OPERATIVE URETHROCYSTOSCOPY

CHAPTER 11

Periurethral injections for intrinsic urethral sphincteric deficiency

Alfred E. Bent

OVERVIEW

The past 25 years have seen a gradual transformation in the use of periurethral bulking agents almost exclusively to the use of collagen.[1,2] The process moved from sclerosing agents to autologous blood, then to polytetrafluoroethylene paste and autologous fat, and now to Contigen (C.R. Bard Inc., Covington, Georgia, USA). Other materials including silicone polymers and autologous tissues are also under investigation.

The approval of Contigen by the United States Food and Drug Administration (FDA) for intrinsic sphincter deficiency (ISD) in the fall of 1993 was the turning point for use of collagen material as a bulking agent, and its use was greatly enhanced when Medicare started reimbursing for the materials and procedure on July 11, 1994.[3] The criteria for use were updated on October 7, 1996[4] (Table 11.1).

The effectiveness reported in studies required to obtain approval of the FDA was 46% cure (63 of 137), and 34% (47 of 137) improved. Although much higher cure rates have been quoted, repeat injections may be required for maximal benefit. The collagen has a tissue life of 3–19 months, at which time the effect at the bladder neck can be expected to diminish and repeat injection is required.

PREOPERATIVE CRITERIA FOR COLLAGEN

Collagen is indicated for the patient with ISD and immobility of the bladder neck. The Medicare guidelines currently state that collagen may be used in patients who have a negative skin test result observed over 4 weeks, an abdominal leak point pressure (LPP) of less than 100 cm H_2O with a minimum of 150 ml in the bladder, and no urethral hypermobility. The physician must have training in cystoscopy and must have completed a collagen implant training pro-

Table 11.1 Medicare guidelines for collagen injection

A. July 11, 1994
   Negative skin test
   Bladder neck hypomobility
   Abdominal leak point pressure less than 65 cm H_2O (with a minimum of 150 ml in the bladder)
   Incontinence without improvement for 12 months or longer
   No more than five injections allowed

B. October 7, 1996 (changes are listed)
   Abdominal leak point pressure less than 100 cm H_2O
   Number of injections unlimited if improvement documented
   Requirement for 12 months' observation showing no improvement of incontinence removed

Table 11.2 Contraindications to collagen injection

Absolute contraindications
  Positive skin test
  Hypersensitivity to collagen material
  History of severe allergy or anaphylaxis
  Patients undergoing desensitization to meat products
  Active urinary tract infection

Relative contraindications
  Detrusor hyperreflexia
  Low compliance bladder
  Vesicoureteral reflux
  Bladder capacity less than 125 ml
  Residual urine determination greater than 250 ml
  Patients with connective tissue disorders

gram. Previous statements were altered in that there is no limit to the number of injections as long as the patient continues to show documented response to therapy. The duration of incontinence at initiation of therapy is not specified, nor does conservative therapy have to be tried before collagen injections. Studies are ongoing to determine the effectiveness of collagen injections in patients with bladder neck hypermobility, and in those with LPP in excess of 100 cm H_2O.

Difficulties arise with these guidelines in that the technique for determining the LPP is not described as the patient position and bladder volume are not stipulated, and yet these parameters have been shown to affect the LPP results.[5] Moreover, hypermobility of the urethra is not described, nor is the method to determine it specified. Contraindications to injection include active urinary tract infection, small bladder capacity (<125 ml), and hypersensitivity to collagen material (Table 11.2).

The work-up should include history and physical examination, urinalysis and culture, postvoid residual urine determination, voiding diary, cystometrogram, Q-tip test or imaging of bladder neck mobility, LPP, urethral closure pressure profiles, and cystourethroscopy (Table 11.3). The criteria for diagnosing ISD vary by center,

Table 11.3 Pretreatment evaluation

History and physical examination
Urinalysis and/or culture
Residual urine determination
Voiding diary
Cystometrography
Q-tip test or imaging for bladder neck mobility
Abdominal leak point pressure estimation
Cystourethroscopy

Table 11.4 Pretreatment patient counseling (informed consent)

Allergic or autoimmune reaction
Urinary tract infection
Bleeding
Pain with injection
Use of local anesthetic
Voiding difficulty
Need to self-catheterize
Success rates
Repeat injections

but findings should include a number of the following to indicate or suggest poor urethral resistance: clinically severe stress incontinence, positive supine empty stress test, urethral closure pressure <20 cm H_2O in the sitting full position, LPP <65 cm H_2O performed in the sitting position with 150–200 ml in the bladder, and endoscopic visualization of impaired bladder neck function (see Chapter 5). The criteria for diagnosing immobility of the bladder neck would include a straining Q-tip test of less than 30–40°, vertical descent of the bladder neck of less than 2 cm during stress cystography or ultrasonographic visualization, type III incontinence on cystography, or impaired mobility of the bladder neck on video studies.[6] The patient signs an informed consent before injection (Table 11.4).

PERIURETHRAL TECHNIQUE

The injection can be performed in the outpatient setting. Local anesthetic is injected lateral to the urethral meatus. The panendoscope or urethroscope (0° lens works best) is situated near the open bladder neck after emptying the bladder (Fig. 11.1). The periurethral collagen needle is introduced close to and parallel to the urethra (Fig. 11.2). The correct location is 0.5–1 cm distal to the bladder neck and can be confirmed by moving or jiggling the needle. A test injection of a small amount of indigo carmine-stained 1% xylocaine is made, and the location of bulging into the urethral mucosal lining confirmed. The collagen material is then injected at the selected site, in order to bulge the urethral mucosa into the midline and partially occlude the urethrovesical junction (UVJ) or bladder neck. The procedure is repeated on the opposite side, until the UVJ is mostly occluded (Fig. 11.3) (Plates 8.1–8.4). The patient is asked to cough, and then stands and coughs. She attempts to void, and then self-catheterizes for residual urine.

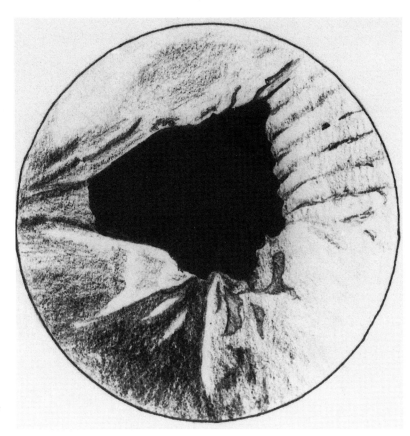

Fig. 11.1 Open bladder neck. The urethrovesical junction is visualized just before collagen injection, using a 0 or 12° telescope

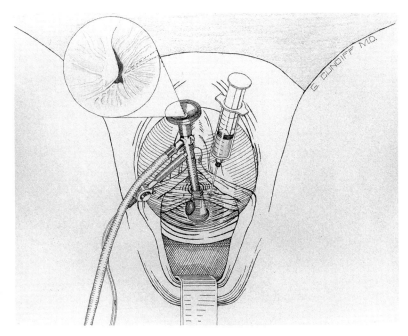

Fig. 11.2 Periurethral collagen injection. The endoscope is in position in the urethra, and is positioned distal to the bladder neck. The periurethral injection needle is advanced alongside the urethroscope. After the site for injection has been determined by injection of indigo carmine-stained local anesthetic, the collagen is placed

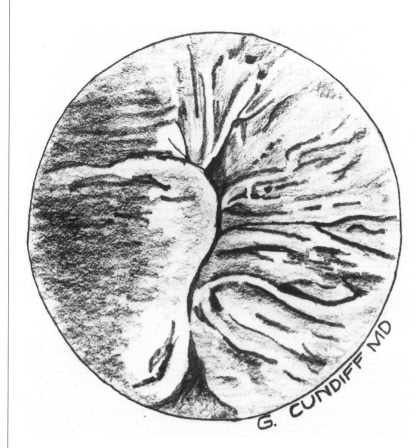

Fig. 11.3 Completed periurethral injection of collagen. Injection of collagen is completed by periurethral technique, and the bladder neck is now closed

TRANSURETHRAL TECHNIQUE

The procedure can be performed in the outpatient setting. The best sheath is one with minimal or no beaking, size 19–21F, and one that can accommodate a transurethral 22 or 23g injection needle as well as the telescope. A 12 or 30° telescope is optimal. Benzocaine 20% can be applied topically to the urethral meatus and urethra. A bladder pillar block may be administered[7] or a small amount of 1% xylocaine may be injected into the urethral mucosa near the collagen injection site to afford analgesia. The endoscope is passed into the bladder and the bladder contents are drained. The collagen material is advanced through the needle until it is visualized at the needle tip. The endoscope is withdrawn from the bladder with the needle protected by the sheath. A site 1–1.5 cm distal to the bladder neck is selected at the 3 o'clock location and the injection needle advanced just under the surface of the urethral mucosa. Some surgeons prefer the bevel to face the lumen, and others contend it should be directed away from the urethral lumen. The collagen is deposited slowly until the bulge in the mucosa partially occludes the bladder neck. Visualization becomes difficult at this point, but the injection should be continued

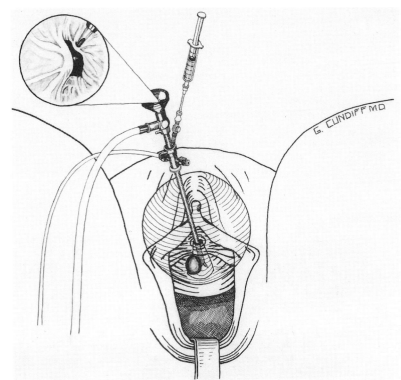

Fig. 11.4 Transurethral collagen injection. The endoscope is held at the bladder neck, and somewhat distal, to observe the needle being passed to the bladder neck tissues. A location 1 cm distal to the bladder neck area is selected, and the collagen is introduced at the 3 and 9 o'clock positions

as long as bulging continues. It is preferred not to pass the endoscope through the bladder neck again, once the first side has been done. The procedure is repeated on the opposite site at the 9 o'clock position (Fig. 11.4). Additional location sites may be required, but usually a total of 5–7.5 ml of collagen material is injected. The needle puncture sites seal rapidly and minimal collagen escapes by this route (Plates 8.5–8.12).

In the author's experience most patients receiving periurethral collagen have been unable to void adequately for 6–24 hours, so all are instructed in self-catheterization several days before the injection. Patients receiving transurethral collagen are much more likely to void, and are offered the opportunity to wait on site for a few hours to ensure voiding is normal. Prophylaxis is given for 2–3 days. Patients are contacted by phone the next day to ensure voiding is normal. The first office follow-up is at 1 month. Early failures may be retreated as early as 1 month. If three injections make no difference in symptoms, further injections are not offered (Table 11.5).

Common complications include urinary retention, urinary tract infection, and recurrent or persistent incontinence. Prolapse of the injected collagen has also been described, although this is a rare complication[8] (Plates 8.13 and 8.14).

Table 11.5 Postinjection management

Instruct in self-catheterization before the injection
Antibiotic prophylaxis for 2–3 days
Allow to void and perform self-catheterization for residual urine
If unable to do self-catheterization, and unable to void, wait in clinic a few hours to ensure adequate voiding
Phone contact day after injection to assess voiding adequacy
Follow-up at 1 month, 3 months, and then yearly
Consider reinjection for failures at 6 weeks
Repeat injections as needed for successful procedures

REFERENCES

1. Appell RA, Winter JC. Periurethral bulking agents. In Ostergard DR, Bent AE (eds) *Urogynecology and Urodynamics: Theory and Practice*, 4th edn. Baltimore: Williams and Wilkins, 1996: 623–9.
2. Appell RA. Periurethral injections. In Hurt WG (ed.) *Urogynecologic Surgery*. Gaithersburg: Aspen, 1992: 139–45.
3. Department of Health and Human Services. *Medicare Coverage Issues Manual: Incontinence Control Devices*. Health Care Financing Administration, Transmittal no. 70, Section 65–9, June 1994.
4. Department of Health and Human Services. *Medicare Coverage Issues Manual: Incontinence Control Devices*. Healthcare Financing Administration, Transmittal no. 89, Section 65–9, September 1996.
5. Theofrastus JP, Cundiff GW, Harris RL, Bump RC. The effect of increasing vesical volume on Valsalva leak point pressures in women with genuine stress incontinence. *Obstet Gynecol* 1996; **87**: 711–14.
6. Bent AE. Periurethral collagen injections. *Operative Techniques in Gynecologic Surgery* 1997; **2**: 51–5.
7. Ostergard DR. Bladder pillar block anesthesia for urethral dilatation in women. *Am J Obstet Gynecol* 1980; **136**: 187–8.
8. Harris RL, Cundiff GW, Coates KW, Addison WA, Bump RC. Urethral prolapse after collagen injection. *Am J Obstet Gynecol* (in press).

CHAPTER 12

Endoscopic photography of bladder and urethra

Alfred E. Bent

INTRODUCTION

Endoscopic imaging allows viewing and recording of normal anatomy, pathology, and endoscopic procedures. Recording may be used in patient education before operation, at the time of the procedure, or after operation as a review of findings. Video imaging provides continuous monitoring for direct hands-on teaching of residents and other physicians. Information preserved in many formats may be used in lecture situations, video presentations, and contributions to scientific and clinical literature. The continuous advances in technology offer the clinician and teacher a wide range of available modalities depending on the quality of image required. Quality slides and prints were previously available through 35-mm camera and lens systems. Virtually all modern systems depend on quality video projection with several ways in which to capture a permanent slide or print.

TELESCOPIC LENS

Chapter 2 discussed preferred systems including telescopic lenses, sheaths, and light sources. A standard cystoscope and hysteroscope telescope lens is 4 mm. The new micro-hysteroscopes and micro-laparoscopes are 2–3 mm in diameter. A lens with a larger diameter delivers a larger picture on the monitor and delivers more light. The conventional lens system was developed by Nitze in 1879, and 1966 brought the introduction of the Hopkins rod lens system, in which special glass rods with optically finished ends replaced the old lens system. A second generation of the rod lens system further advanced the resolution, brightness, contrast, and field of view. The objective or distal lens creates an image at the operative site, and the ocular or proximal lens magnifies the image. Flexible endoscopes were developed to accommodate natural curves of internal body organs. They transmit light through optical glass fibers, but these do not offer the clarity and light-carrying capacity of rod-shaped lenses.

FIBEROPTIC LIGHT CABLES

Light cables are available in various lengths from 6 to 12 feet, and in different diameters from 3.5 to 4.8 mm. The longer the fiberoptic light cable, the less light it delivers, with approximately 10% light loss for every foot of cable over 6 feet. A 6–9-foot cable is adequate for good video. The quantity of light delivery improves in direct proportion to the thickness of the cable. However, it is more important to match the telescopic lens size with the fiberoptic light cable, i.e. a hysteroscope and cystoscope generally perform best with a 3.5-mm diameter cable versus a 4.8-mm cable, which is designed for a 10-mm laparoscope. The light transmission of a fiberoptic cable can be checked by holding one end to a light, and viewing the other end for fiber damage. Black dots or gray areas indicate damage, and replacement should be made if over 20% of the fibers are damaged.

LIGHT SOURCE

A halogen 150-watt lamp is available as an adequate light source for a procedure without video. It requires a 30-second warm-up time and a 5-minute cool-down time. Frequent on and off cycling can shorten bulb life, and the lamp loses brightness with time. Although less expensive than xenon, it is not as bright. When using video, a xenon light is much brighter and more effective. A xenon system produces high intensity white light and high color temperature which corresponds to sunlight. It responds immediately when turned on, and the lamp gradually loses brightness over time, but it is not affected by on and off cycling. A standard 175-watt xenon lamp may cost from $2000 to $4000. More expensive models, often used in the operating room, permit light intensity adjustment manually or automatically and have a display of lamp-hours. A 300-watt xenon lamp is available as top of the line equipment, but most documentation can be done with the 175-watt system.

VIDEO CAMERA

The video camera has transformed the viewing process from one of isolation to all those in the endoscopic area, including patient, allied health personnel, and physicians. No longer must the operator bend at an uncomfortable angle in order to see all areas of the bladder adequately, and the results are available immediately.

The endoscopic video camera consists of a small camera head, a camera head cable, and a camera processor. The camera head contains a lens and one to three light-sensitive imaging chips called charged couple devices (CCDs). An adapter (endocoupler) connects the camera head to the eyepiece of a scope, and it contains optical lenses and the focusing adjustment. Endocouplers come in focal lengths of different size, including 25, 30, 38, and 50 mm. The longer the focal length, the larger the picture on the monitor. However, the longer the focal length (e.g. 25 versus 50 mm) the greater the light quantity needed to produce a good video image on the monitor. If the image size is doubled, four times the quantity of light will be needed to produce a good video image. A parfocal zoom lens has a focal length of 25–50 mm. It eliminates the need to purchase several differently sized endocouplers. The integrated zoom optics eliminates the need to refocus when magnifying the image. The camera head cable connects the camera head to the camera processor. The cable end plug may be a card edge connector, which allows excellent signal transfer and is easy to clean, or it may be a round-end connector, which must be covered with a soaking cap before disinfecting in solution.

The camera processor or camera control unit (CCU) houses the camera's operating controls including power switch, white-balance, and a light boost or 'gain' to compensate for low light conditions. Some cameras have a microprocessor-controlled electronic autoshutter that controls the camera's shutter speed to adjust to varying light levels.

The camera lens focuses the image on the camera CCDs, and each CCD has linear rows of light-sensitive silicon cells (pixels), the number of which affects the color and resolution of the video image. Each pixel generates electrical activity in proportion to the amount of light hitting it. The signal is generated on a line-by-line basis, through a process called scanning.

ONE-CHIP VERSUS THREE-CHIP CAMERA

Medical video cameras are available as one or three video chips. The key differences between a one-chip and three-chip cameras are color and resolution. It is important to understand some of the basic video terms and features of each camera in order to understand their differences. Single-chip cameras have one CCD to reproduce color and create an image. They provide an excellent image and are more compact and less expensive than three-chip cameras. A three-chip camera has a prism which refracts the light into the three primary colors (red, green, blue). Each chip picks up one color, providing a better quality image at considerable expense.

RESOLUTION

Resolution is the ability of a video camera to resolve detail. Resolution is described as the number of black and white lines per inch that can be seen as distinct lines. Horizontal resolution is measured by the number of vertically oriented alternating black and white lines that can be seen by an observer. Single-chip cameras have 300–450 lines of horizontal resolution, and three-chip cameras have as many as 750 lines per inch. The higher the number of lines of horizontal resolution, the sharper the image.

LIGHT SENSITIVITY

Light sensitivity is the ability of a camera to make a useable picture in low light. It is measured in lux for a given lens aperture, measured in f-stops. Generally, the lower the lux specification, the better the camera's ability to see in low light conditions.

VIDEO FORMAT

The video signal generated by the camera's CCDs must be processed and transmitted to the monitor. The video signal has three components: chrominance (C), which carries color information; luminance (Y), which carries picture brightness and fine picture detail; and synchronization, which synchronizes the scanning of the image. A composite format (NTSC) is the oldest, but is not as good for the newer high-resolution cameras. The signal is carried in one wire, and all cameras have composite capability even if they are capable of advanced formats. The YC format (or S-VHS) separates chrominance and luminance on two separate wires, and sends the synchronization on one of the wires. It is the best format for one-chip cameras. The RGB format provides outstanding color clarity and quality. The red, green, and blue color signals are carried with their corresponding luminance on separate lines, and synchronization signals are carried on a fourth line. The picture tube in the monitor converts the chrominance, luminance, and synchronization signals into light energy which works across and down the screen, forming 525 horizontal lines, in 1/30th of a second. It is the best format for three-chip cameras and some one-chip cameras. It provides the best color and best detail. All documentation equipment is capable of using RGB format, except the video recorder that still uses YC and composite format.

MONITOR

A camera capable of 700 lines of resolution would be wasted on a monitor with any less resolution. In surgery, a monitor with a 19-inch diagonal screen is popular because it is more clearly seen, although the image is much brighter on a smaller screen, such as a 13-inch size. Thus, for a one-chip camera the monitor should have at least 450 lines of resolution, and ideally the monitor should have 750 lines of resolution for a three-chip camera.

VIDEO CASSETTE RECORDER

As with the other equipment, there are several choices of recording equipment for moving images. The least expensive is VHS (very high speed) at a cost of approximately $500, and which has approximately 240 lines of horizontal resolution. Super-VHS is a more expensive type of tape, but of better quality than the VHS format. Super-VHS recorders have approximately 400 lines of resolution, but can also play or record on VHS tapes. They cost approximately twice as much as VHS recorders. A medical grade S-VHS recorder is also available with double fine slow motion and automatic digital tracking, as well as other features.

VIDEO PRINTER

A video printer (Sony Medical Systems, Montvale, NJ, USA) stores a still image from a video camera and then produces a high-quality print. Multiple split-screen prints of size 4 × 5 inches may be selected, and the basic models have no extra memory, print in 60 seconds, and have 500 lines of resolution. A premium printer at four times the cost can have over 700 lines of horizontal resolution, a four- or eight-frame memory, optional SCSI computer interface, and can print hard copies sized 5 × 8 inches in 30 seconds.

SURGICAL SLIDE MAKER

A surgical slide maker (Surgislide; MedGraphix International Imaging, Rosemont, PA, USA) is available to produce presentation quality 35-mm color slides from standard video signals. Systems may allow up to four pictures in a row without any wait time, or an average of one picture every 6 seconds. The horizontal resolution is 800 lines (when using a high-resolution display monitor), and the preferred video source is RGB with a three-chip video camera. Slides may be produced on quality Kodak film (100EPN), and film and development costs are less than $1 per slide. The drawback for this system is that the whole image exposed to the film is not known until the film is developed. The major advantages are reasonable cost and ability to produce good quality slides.

DIGITAL STILL RECORDER

A digital still recorder (Sony Medical Systems) picks up an endoscopic video image, and assigns an identification number and time stamp. The pictures are displayed on screen in real time, and may be selected and archived for documentation, or they may be erased if the image is not desirable. The horizontal resolution is 500 lines, and pictures are stored on a magneto-optical disk, which can accommodate 100 high-quality images or 1000 low-quality images. Images may be retrieved by the unit or on computer display for sorting and displaying images, as well as adding text and comments. Slides can be made from disk, although these, and the system itself, are expensive. The main advantage of this system is the capability to select the desired images and to erase the others. This is the desired device for publication, teaching, research endeavors, and documentation.

OFFICE SYSTEM

The standard office system for visualization and documentation might consist of the 175-watt office xenon light source, single chip video camera, 13-inch color monitor with 450 lines of resolution, standard VHS video cassette recorder, and basic model video printer. This equipment costs in the range of US $6500–12 000 and can be stored on a portable office medical cart (Fig. 12.1).

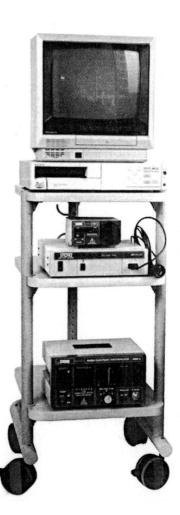

Fig. 12.1 Office medical cart. This portable cart has shelving for the office equipment needed to perform cystourethroscopy with documentation capability. It can be moved to different rooms or locations, and should be locked in a secure area when not in use

Table 12.1 Troubleshooting checklist

Problem	Possible remedy
No power	Plug in all components; turn on power Ensure wall outlets are functional Check fuses where appropriate
No picture	Recheck power on all components Is camera head plugged in? Isolate camera and monitor, and other components in sequence Is light source brightness all the way up? Is fiberoptic cable plugged in all the way? Check monitor, VCR buttons – the connections must correlate with the lines used (Y, A, B, RGB) Check VCR pause button Monitor buttons must be specified for each type of connection Cables may be nonfunctioning, especially old ones
Image not in focus	Focus camera Check camera coupler – detach from scope and aim at wall, and refocus to check camera Look through scope; make sure it is clear and sharp Check camera cable connector Clean scope and camera lenses with 70% isopropyl alcohol; make sure both are dry Check with company representative
Image dark	Check power and connections Check light cable for broken fibers and replace if worn; is it plugged in all the way? Check scope for broken fibers, replace if worn Turn up light intensity of light source Check lamp life (bulb) and replace if old Adjust monitor brightness Clean all lenses; wipe tissue or blood from lens tip Zoom down on object will reduce magnification and reduce the amount of light necessary to view properly Adjust gain to high on new cameras with gain control
Poor color	White balance Readjust monitor with color bar pattern Check knobs on front of monitor Clean scopes Clean camera cable with alcohol and dry connection
Reference	Refer to qualified personnel Video or print the problem seen on the monitor

A state of the art imaging and recording system for research, publication, and teaching should consist of a 300-watt xenon light source with automatic light intensity adjustment, three-chip camera, high-grade monitor with 750 lines of resolution, top of the line S-VHS recorder, premium video printer, and either a surgical slide maker or digital still recorder. Equipment costs range from US $35 000 to $45 000. A good-quality cart should be purchased to hold all the components, with appropriate electrical access, and locking front and back doors. The cart needs to be in a secure area.

CLEANING AND MAINTENANCE

The devices should be turned off after use and wiped clean with a soft cloth dampened with a mild detergent. Strong cleaners must be avoided. The monitor can be cleaned with water. The components can be dried with a soft towel or gauze sponge. All staff need to be inserviced by the company representative in the care and handling of equipment.

TROUBLESHOOTING

A troubleshooting checklist should be kept by the video cart, and access to manuals and industry representatives kept current. The power cords and video cables should be labeled. A guide for problems is shown in Table 12.1.

APPENDIX 1

Normal anatomy of the lower urinary tract

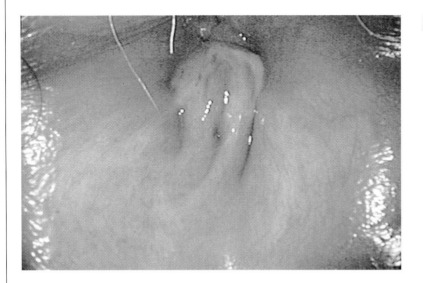

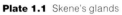
URETHRA

Plate 1.1 Skene's glands

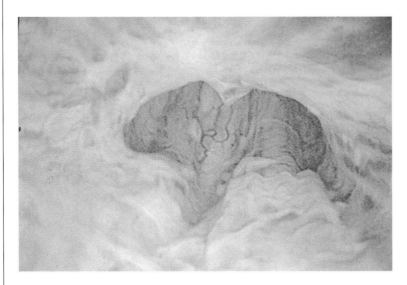

Plate 1.2 Normal urethral color (open to flow)

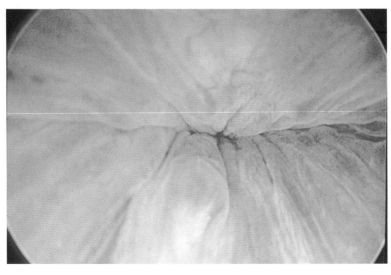

Plate 1.3 Normal urethral coaptation

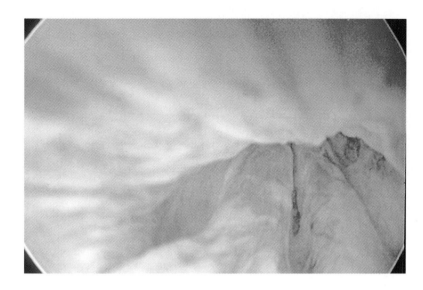

Plate 1.4 Urethral crest

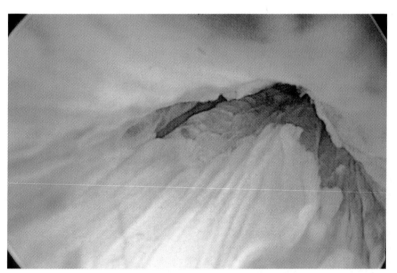

Plate 1.5 Urethral metaplasia

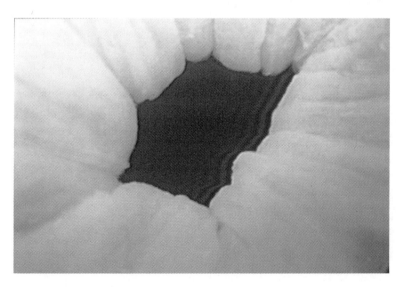

Plate 1.6 Urethrovesical junction, open

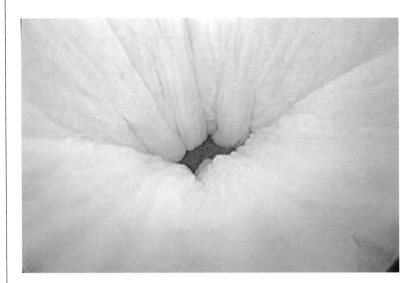

Plate 1.7 Urethrovesical junction, closed

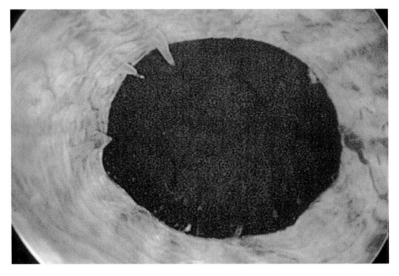

Plate 1.8 Normal voiding

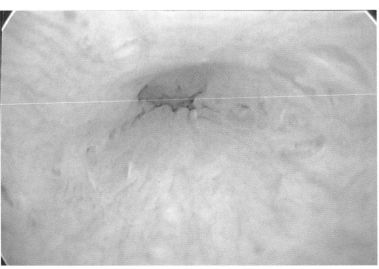

Plate 1.9 Periurethral glands

BLADDER

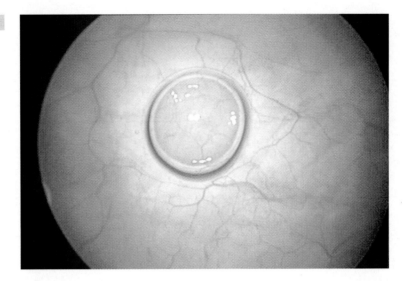

Plate 1.10 Air bubble at 12 o'clock

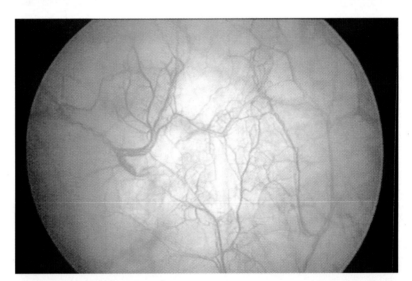

Plate 1.11 Normal mucosa and vascularity

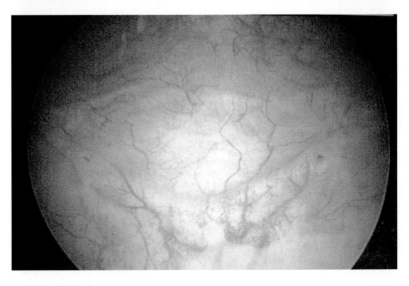

Plate 1.12 Trigone

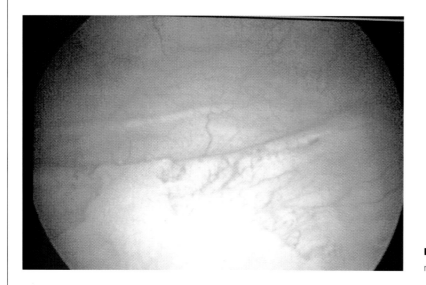

Plate 1.13 Trigone with squamous metaplasia

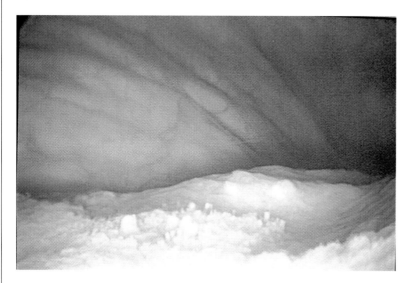

Plate 1.14 Trigone with more pronounced metaplasia

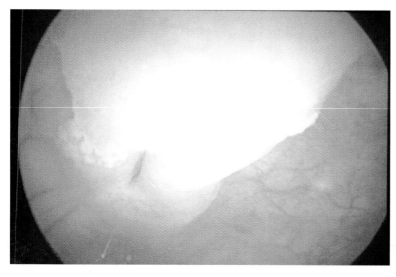

Plate 1.15 Left ureter (with metaplasia)

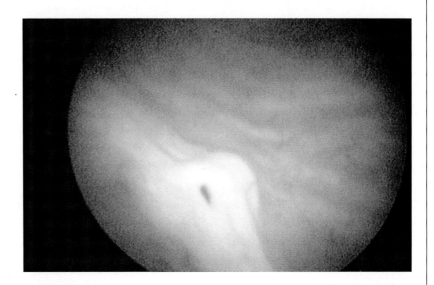

Plate 1.16 Right ureter

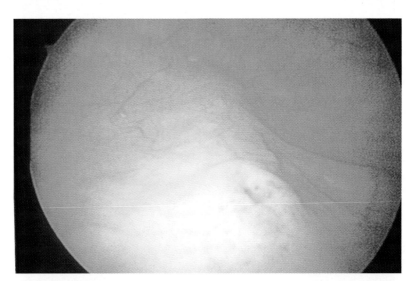

Plate 1.17 Right ureter with efflux
(pyridium-stained urine)

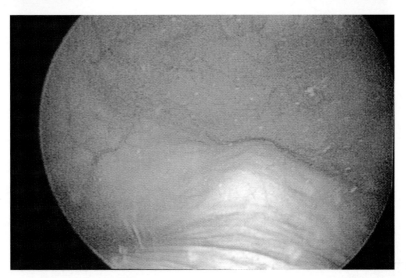

Plate 1.18 Indentation of uterus

Nonpathologic abnormalities of the lower urinary tract

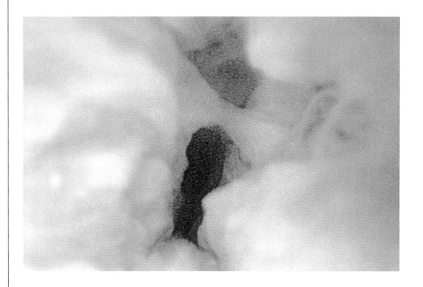

URETHRA

Plate 2.1 Transverse septum in the proximal urethra

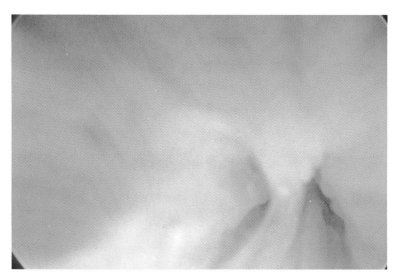

Plate 2.2 Vertical septum in the distal urethra

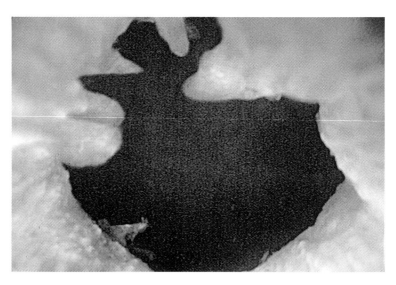

Plate 2.3 Urethrovesical junction fronds

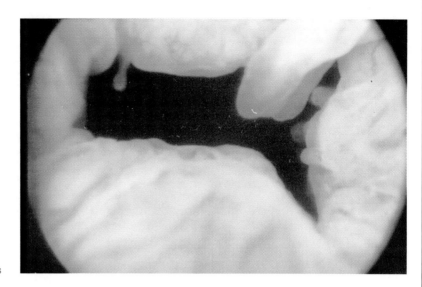

Plate 2.4 Urethrovesical junction fronds

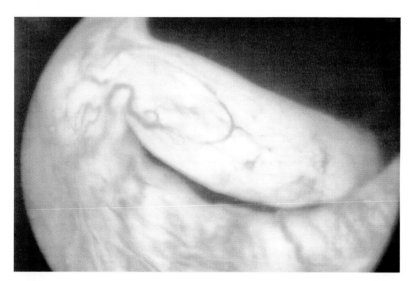

Plate 2.5 Urethral polyp

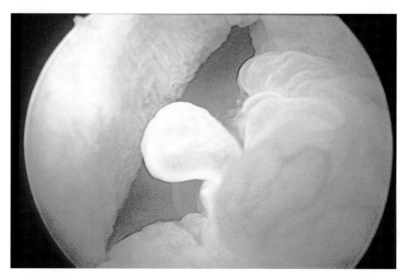

Plate 2.6 Urethral polyp

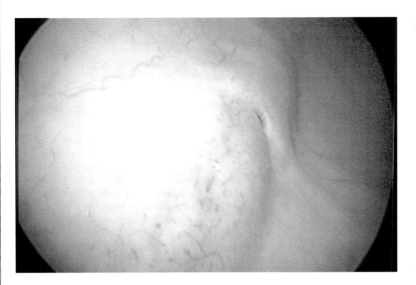

BLADDER

Plate 2.7 Double ureters

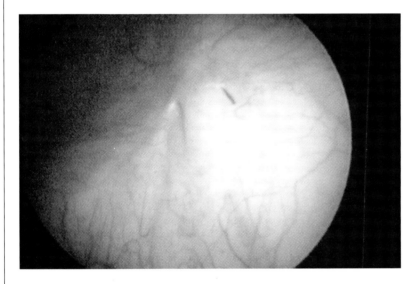

Plate 2.8 Double ureters

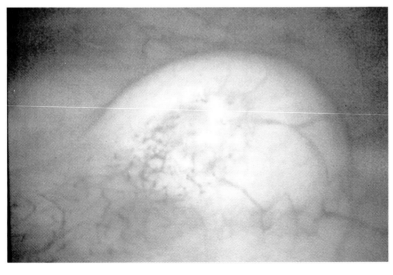

Plate 2.9 Ureterocele

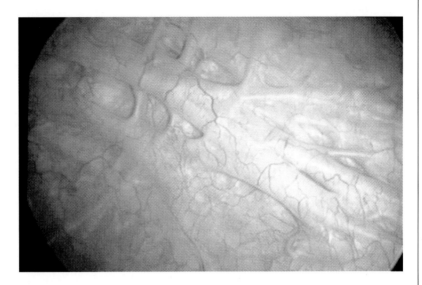

Plate 2.10 Trabeculations, mild

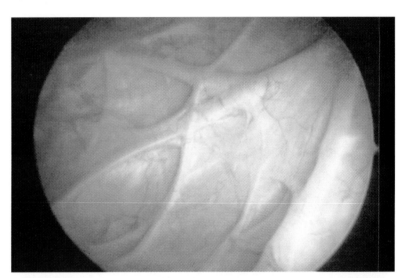

Plate 2.11 Trabeculations, moderate

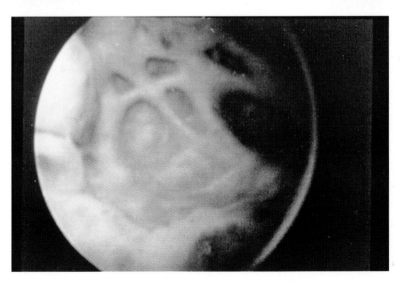

Plate 2.12 Trabeculations, severe

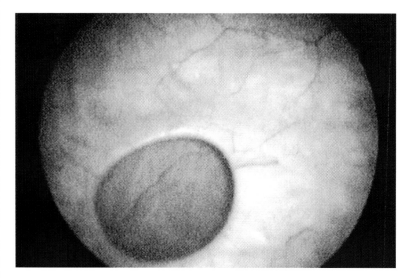

Plate 2.13 Bladder diverticulum

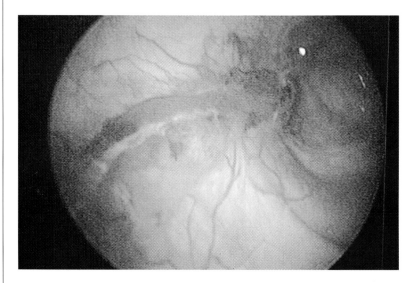

Plate 2.14 Bladder scar in dome (acute)

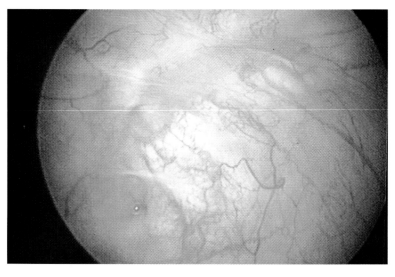

Plate 2.15 Bladder scar in dome (chronic)

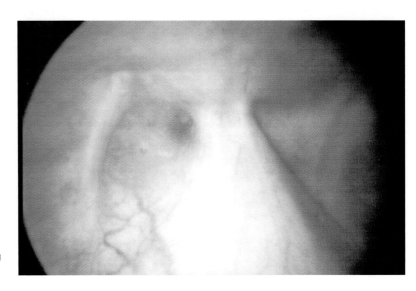

Plate 2.16 Bladder scar status following fistula repair

APPENDIX 3

Inflammatory changes of the lower urinary tract

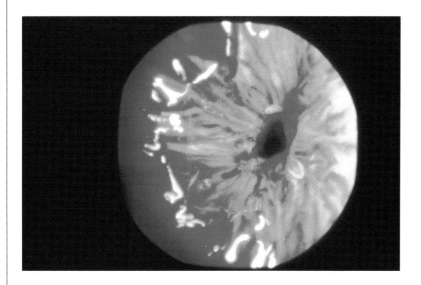

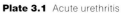

URETHRA

Plate 3.1 Acute urethritis

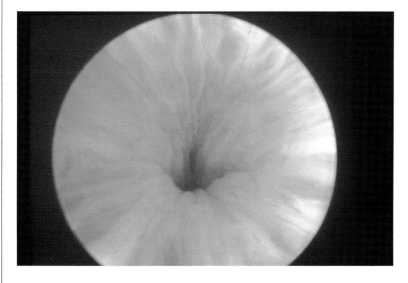

Plate 3.2 Urethral erythema

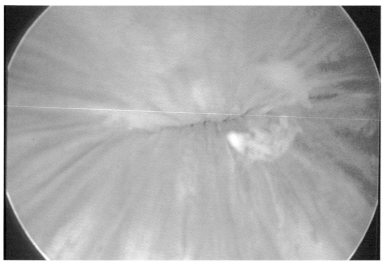

Plate 3.3 Urethral erythema with exudate

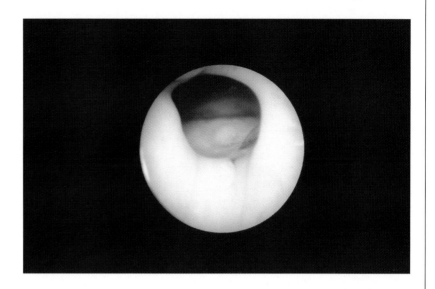

Plate 3.4 Pale hypoestrogenic urethra

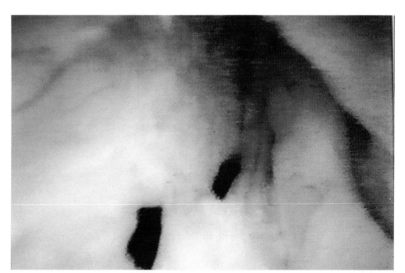

Plate 3.5 Chandelier urethral diverticulum

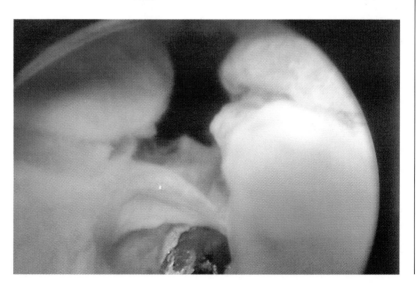

Plate 3.6 Proximal diverticulum with sound in ostium

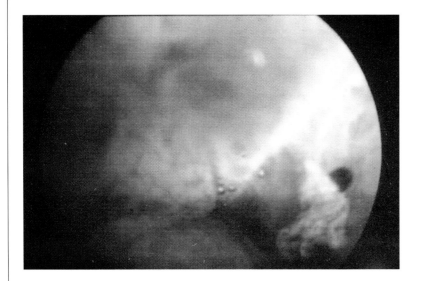

Plate 3.7 Midurethral diverticulum with exudate

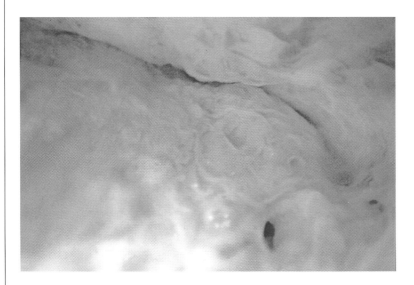

Plate 3.8 Midurethral diverticulum with two ostia

BLADDER – INFLAMMATORY CHANGES

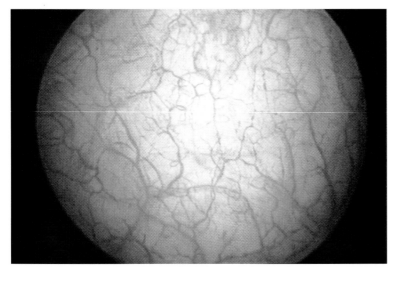

Plate 3.9 Hypervascularity

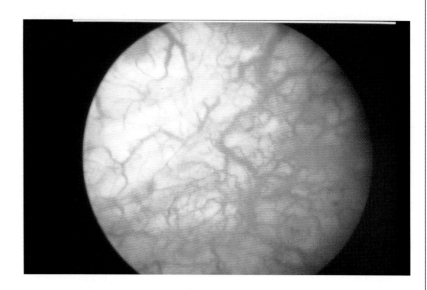

Plate 3.10 Hypervascularity with plaques

Plate 3.11 Dulling of vascular pattern

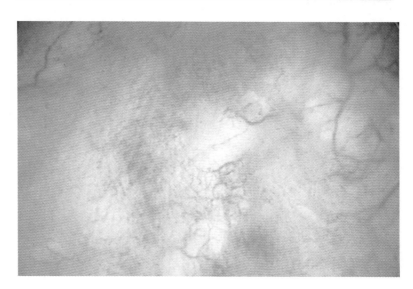

Plate 3.12 Inflammation with edema

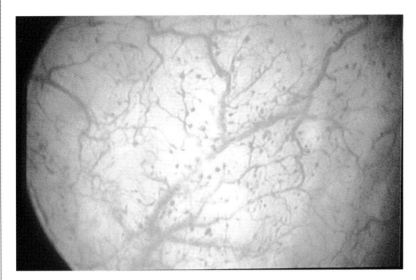

Plate 3.13 Petechial hemorrhages

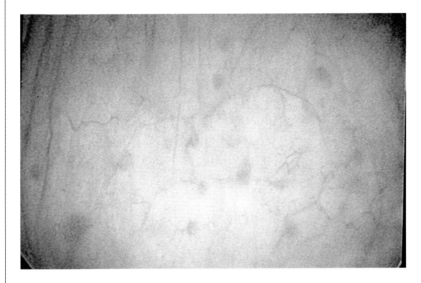

Plate 3.14 Discoid hemorrhages

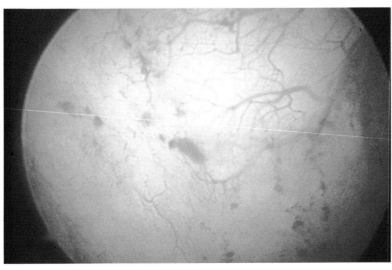

Plate 3.15 Confluent hemorrhages

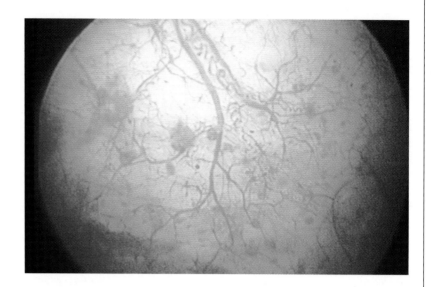

Plate 3.16 Frank hemorrhage

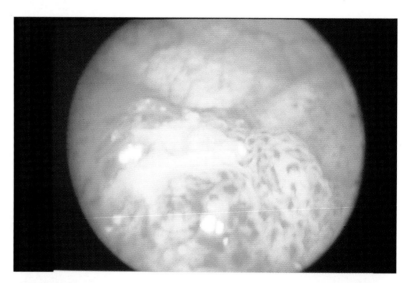

Plate 3.17 Polypoid cystitis

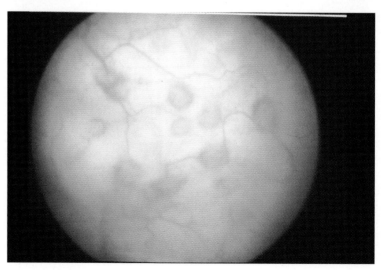

Plate 3.18 Inflammatory bladder plaques

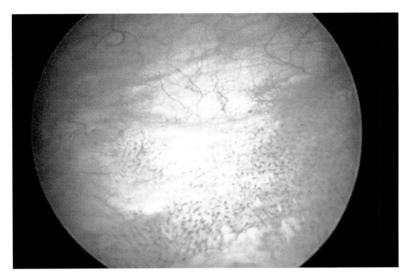

Plate 3.19 Trigonitis, mild

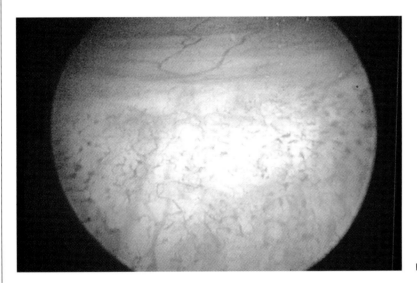

Plate 3.20 Trigonitis, severe

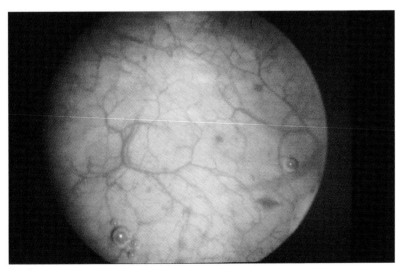

Plate 3.21 Radiation cystitis, chronic

**BLADDER –
INTERSTITIAL CYSTITIS**

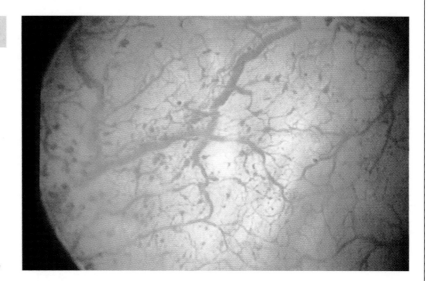

Plate 3.22 Interstitial cystitis, petechiae

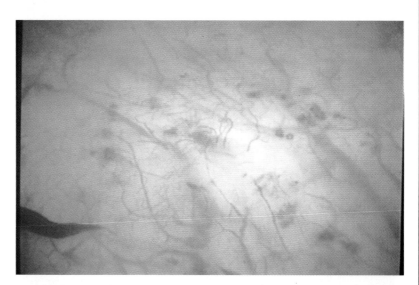

Plate 3.23 Interstitial cystitis, glomerulations

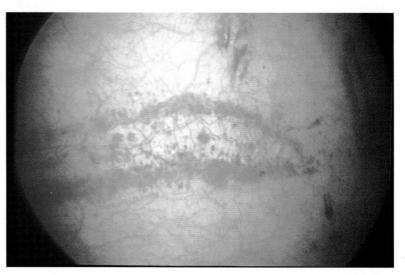

Plate 3.24 Interstitial cystitis, linear hemorrhages

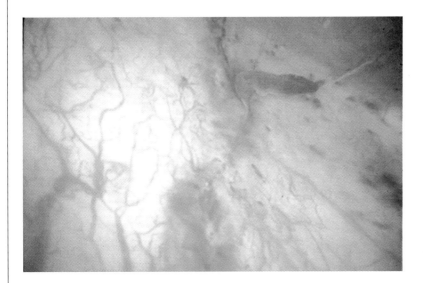

Plate 3.25 Interstitial cystitis, linear hemorrhages with cracks

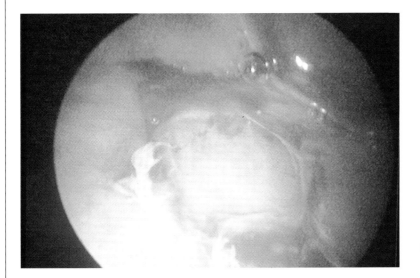

Plate 3.26 Interstitial cystitis, mucosal rupture

Pathology of the lower urinary tract associated with incontinence and pelvic organ prolapse

URETHRA – INTRINSIC SPHINCTERIC DEFICIENCY

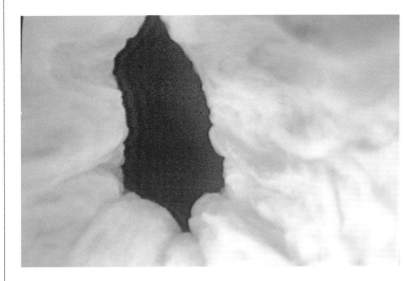

Plate 4.1 Poor coaptation

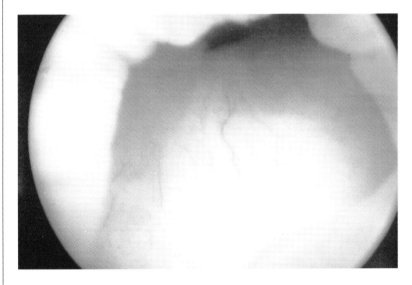

Plate 4.2 Patulous urethra

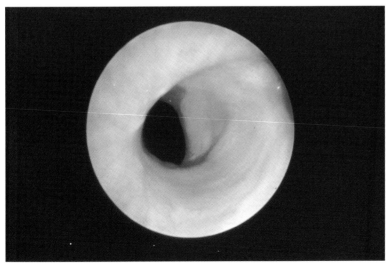

Plate 4.3 Fibrotic urethra

BLADDER – FOREIGN BODIES

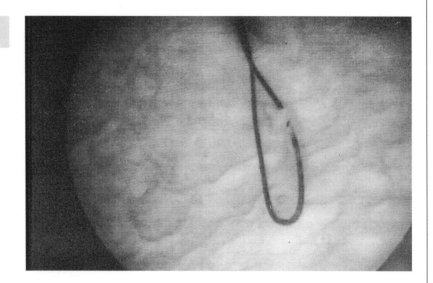

Plate 4.4 Intravesical suture

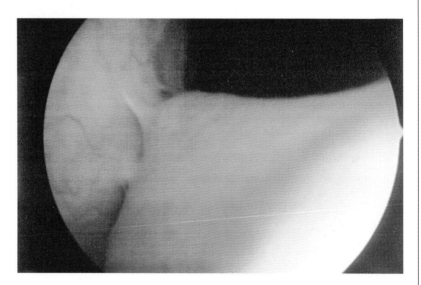

Plate 4.5 Through-and-through suture

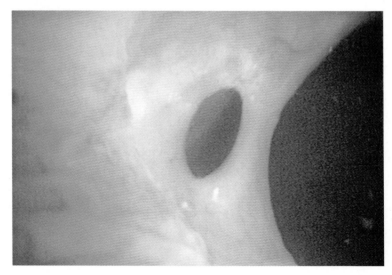

Plate 4.6 Epithelialized suture

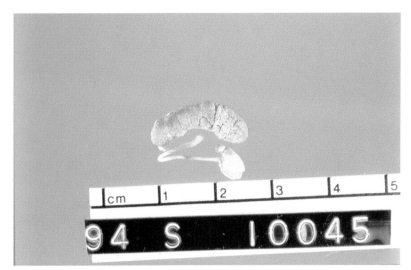

Plate 4.7 Suture lithiasis

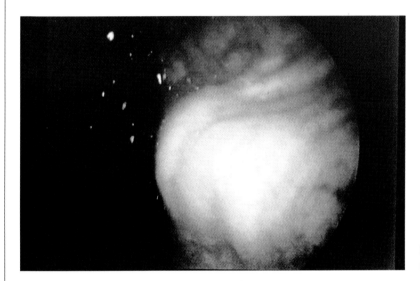

Plate 4.8 Stamey bolster at urethrovesical junction

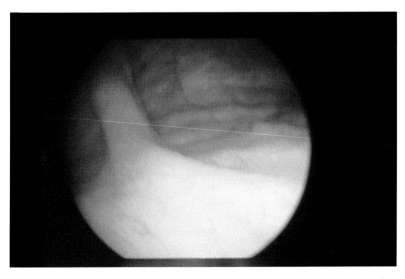

Plate 4.9 Intravesical sling

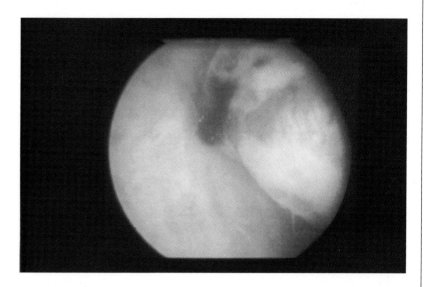

Plate 4.10 Bladder lithiasis

BLADDER – SUPPORT DEFECTS

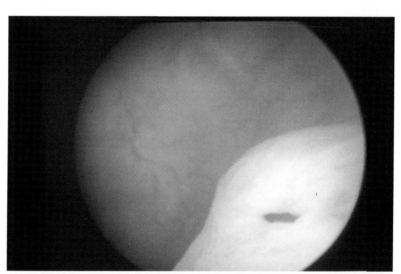

Plate 4.11 Right paravaginal defect

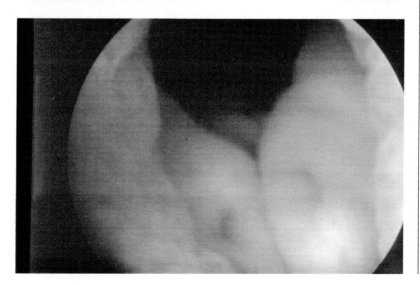

Plate 4.12 Bilateral paravaginal defect

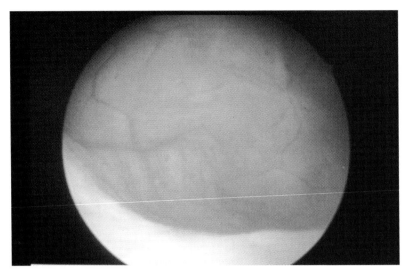

Plate 4.13 Midline cystocele

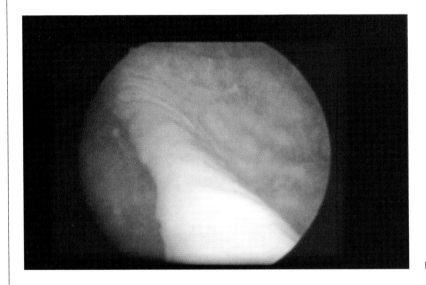

Plate 4.14 Right and midline defect

Mucosal abnormalities of the lower urinary tract associated with hematuria

URETHRA

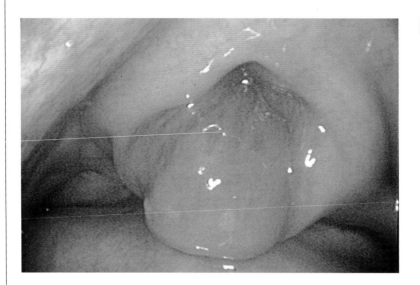

Plate 5.1 Urethral caruncle

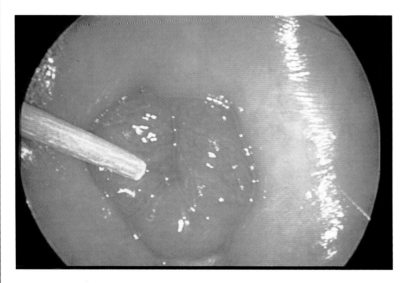

Plate 5.2 Urethral prolapse

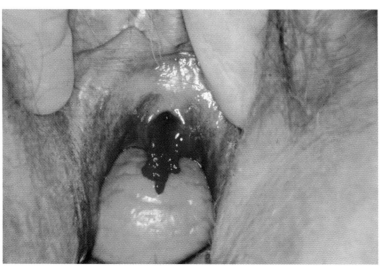

Plate 5.3 Prolapsed urethral polyp

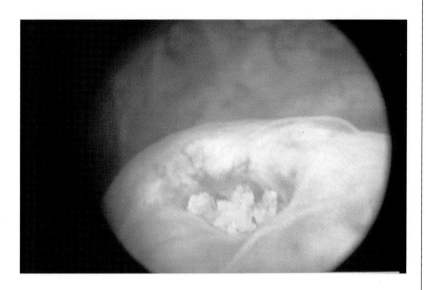

Plate 5.4 Ureteral lithiasis

BLADDER – BENIGN NEOPLASMS

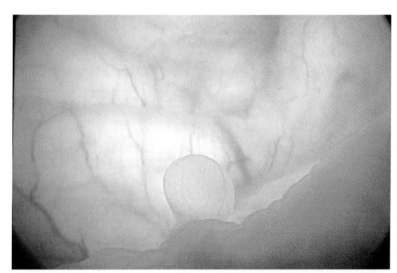

Plate 5.5 Cystitis cystica

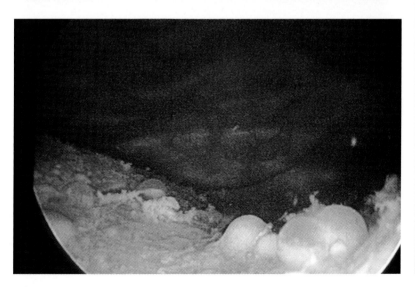

Plate 5.6 Cystitis cystica with liquefaction

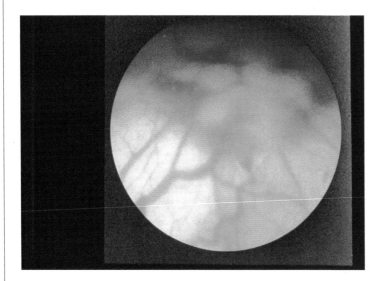

Plate 5.7 Cystitis glandularis

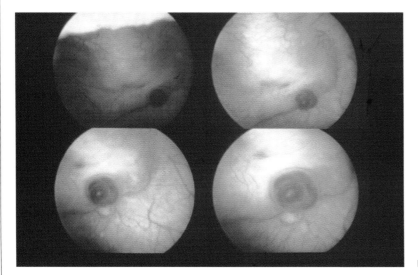

Plate 5.8 Intravesical endometriosis

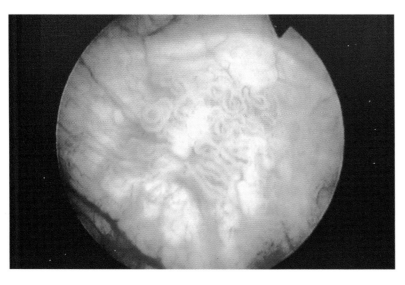

Plate 5.9 Transitional cell papilloma

BLADDER – MALIGNANT NEOPLASMS

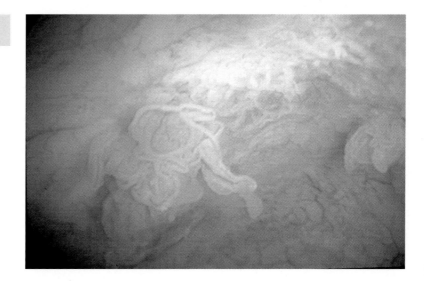

Plate 5.10 Papillary transitional cell carcinoma

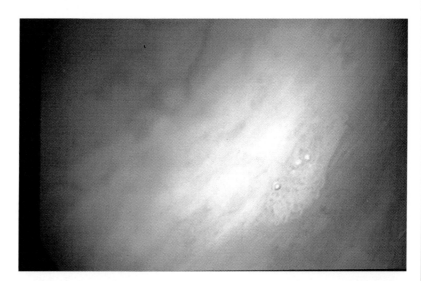

Plate 5.11 Flat transitional cell carcinoma

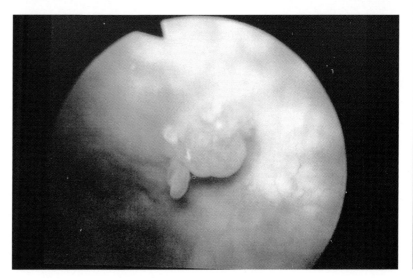

Plate 5.12 Polypoid transitional cell carcinoma

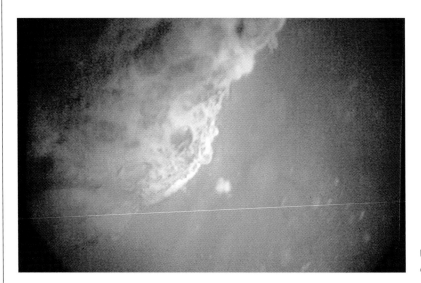

Plate 5.13 Grade 3 invasive transitional cell carcinoma

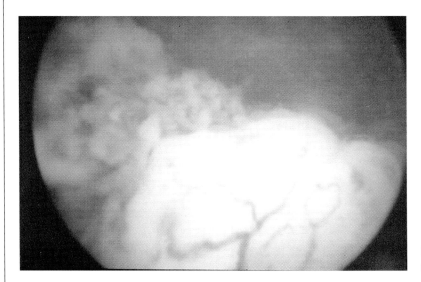

Plate 5.14 Metastatic cervical carcinoma

APPENDIX 6

Fistulas of the lower urinary tract

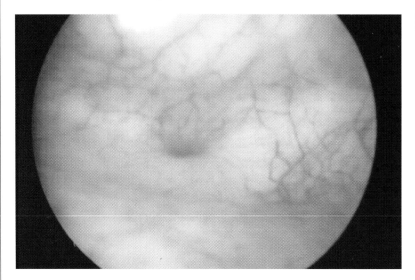

BLADDER

Plate 6.1 Supratrigonal vesicovaginal fistula

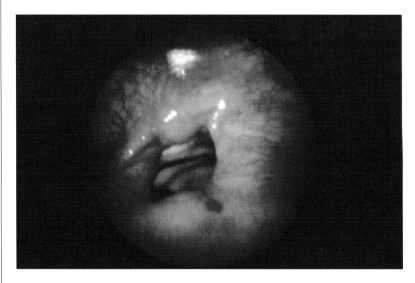

Plate 6.2 Vesicovaginal fistula, vesical ostia

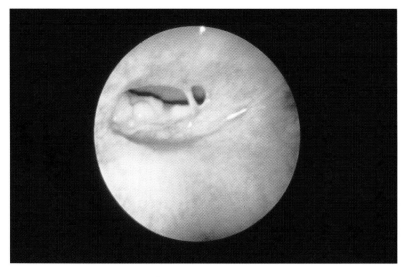

Plate 6.3 Vesicovaginal fistula, vaginal ostia

URETHRA

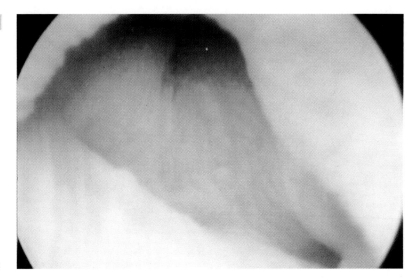

Plate 6.4 Proximal urethrovaginal fistula

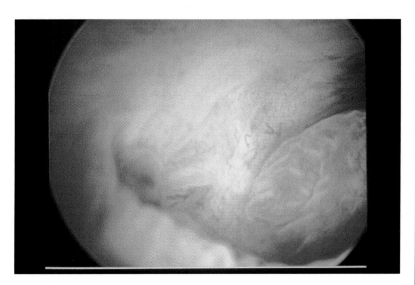

Plate 6.5 Distal urethrovaginal fistula with loss of coaptation

APPENDIX 7

Operative
cystoscopy

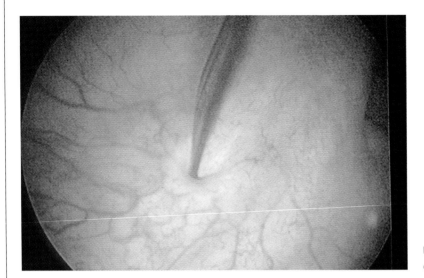

Plate 7.1 Ureteral efflux with indigo carmine-stained urine

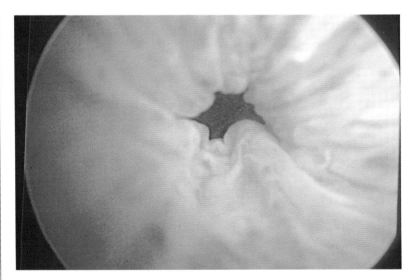

Plate 7.2 Intraoperative assessment of urethrovesical junction, sling relaxed

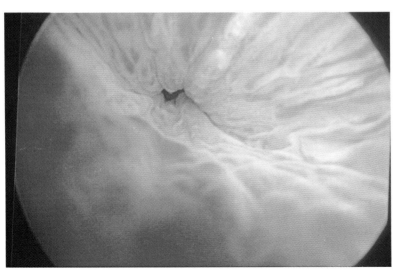

Plate 7.3 Intraoperative assessment of urethrovesical junction, sling elevated

APPENDIX 8

Periurethral injections

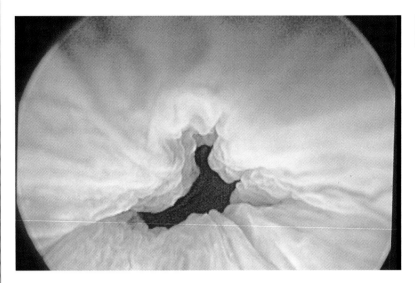

PERIURETHRAL APPROACH

Plate 8.1 Open urethrovesical junction

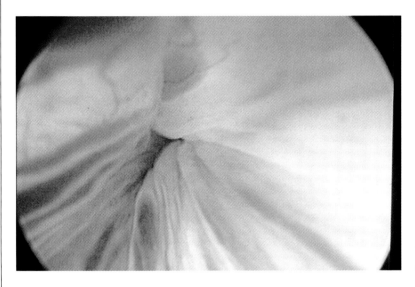

Plate 8.2 Injection in left periurethral space

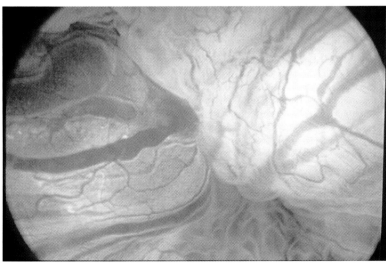

Plate 8.3 Injection in right periurethral space

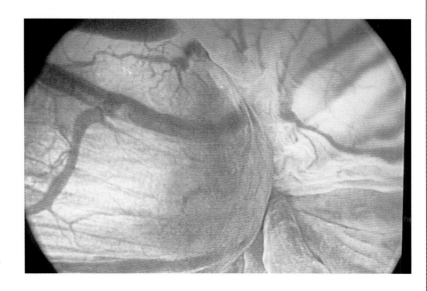

Plate 8.4 Coaptation at completion of injection

TRANSURETHRAL APPROACH

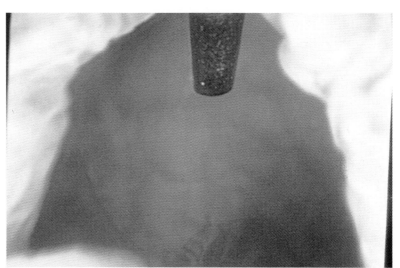

Plate 8.5 Injection needle advanced into field

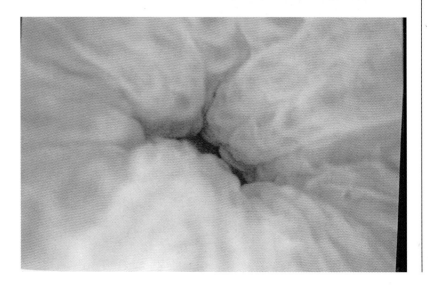

Plate 8.6 Open urethrovesical junction

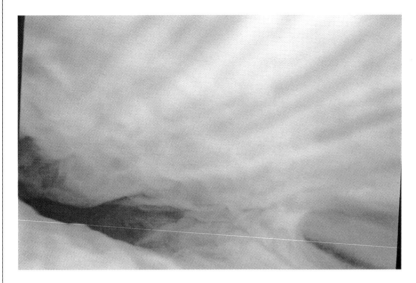

Plate 8.7 Needle inserted at 3 o'clock

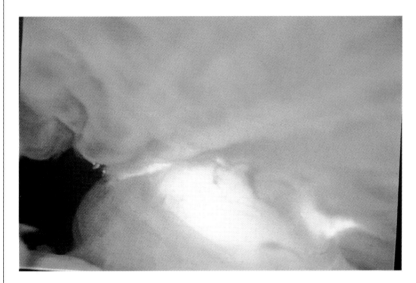

Plate 8.8 Collagen injected on left

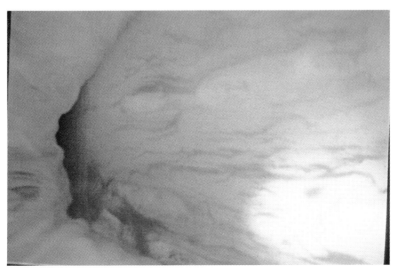

Plate 8.9 Coaptation on left

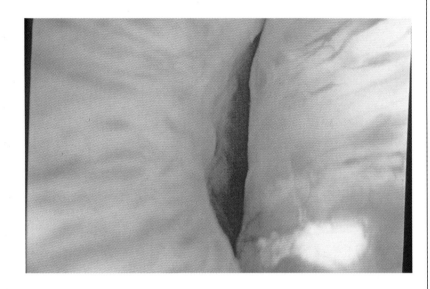

Plate 8.10 Collagen injected on right

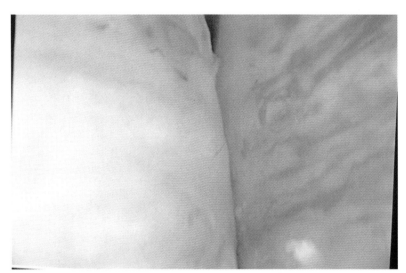

Plate 8.11 Complete coaptation after injection

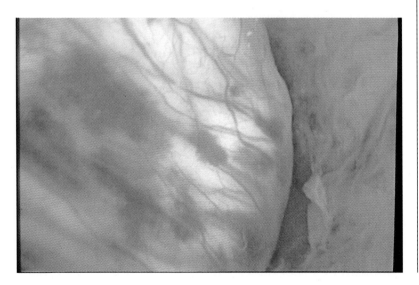

Plate 8.12 Status at 2 months postinjection

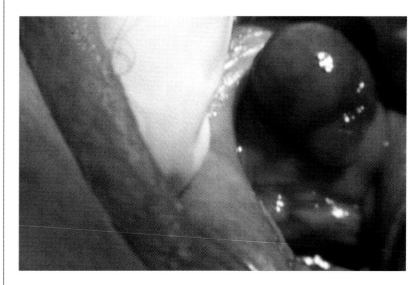

Plate 8.13 Prolapsed injection site

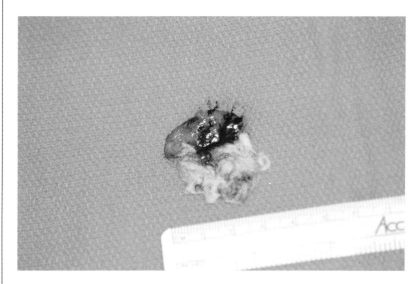

Plate 8.14 Prolapsed injection specimen

Index

INDEX